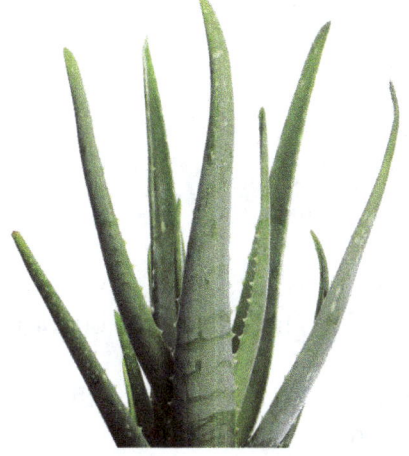

This book is dedicated to my mother and father who have helped me through many difficult times, and to Maxine who showed me how great Aloe vera really is.

I would also love to thank Boogie a great chef who helped me design the food displays throughout the book and made them look so great in the photos - my sincerest appreciation.

Best wishes

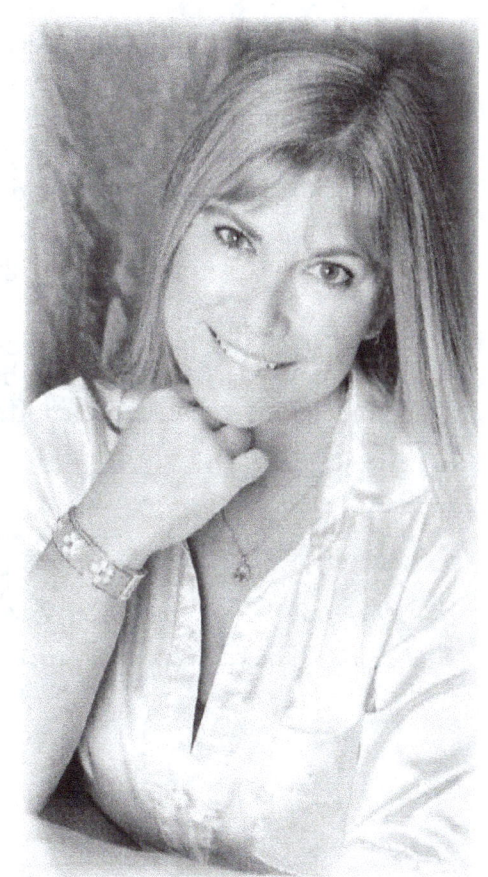

Angela Andrews was born in Victoria, Australia, in 1961. At the age of nineteen she became a fulltime model and actress. Her career spanned fifteen years and she worked on many commercials, movies, mini-series and television shows.

Angie successfully completed a writing course at the Australian College of Journalism in Sydney, in 1996.

Her first four children's books, on *Stranger Danger and Relative and Friendly Danger* were published in 1996.

She is now a distinguished member of the International Poet Society, winning an international award in 2008 for her excellence in poetry for her book, *Aussie Moments*.

The latest title *The Adventures of the Nature Family* was completed in May 2009.

www.angiessmartbooks.com

ENDORSEMENT

Re: Endorsement of "Cookin for Cures"

My name is Horace P. Guerra, IV, MD, founder, owner, and president of International Healing and Hyperbaric, Ltd. (IHH) headquartered out of Las Vegas, NV.

I have tried Angela's recipes, and I am pleased with the results. After ditching the burgers, French fries, pizza and all that processed junk we are accustomed to here in the states, these recipes have been a means of detoxifying the body and getting it back in harmony with the rest of my life. The result is more resilient skin, better energy, more rapid healing, etc. Not to mention, the weight loss has been a nice additive feature

The mysterious powers of *Aloe vera* defies common logic, but it is there. *Aloe vera* has a long association with herbalist medicine, although it is not known exactly when its medical applications were first discovered. Early records of *Aloe vera* use appear in the Ebers Papyrus from 16th century BCE, in both Dioscorides' *De Materia Medica* and Pliny the Elder's *Natural History* written in the mid-first century CE along with the *Juliana Anicia Codex* produced in 512 CE. While this may not mean much to you, this illustrates how long this plant has been recognized as having beneficial effects on the human body.

A recent review (2007) concludes that cumulative evidence supports the use of *Aloe vera* for the healing of first to second degree burns. In addition to topical use in wound or burn healing, internal intake of *Aloe vera* has been linked with improved blood glucose levels in diabetics, and with lower blood lipids in hyperlipidemic patients. Anything that brings down average blood glucose levels and the harmful lipid levels that contribute to coronary artery disease and end organ damage has got to be good in terms of adding to longevity and quality of life.

My sincerest "thank you" to Angela Andrews and her amazing book of healing and appetizing meals. For that I can be thankful for having a more energetic, disease free and much longer than expected life.

Here's to your health!
Sincerely,

Horace P. Guerra, IV, MD
Horace P. Guerra, IV, MD, MPH

CONTENTS

The Big Change

Herbs and their Impressive Use

How to grow your Aloe vera plant

Aloe vera Juice

Drinks

Smoothies

Entrees and soups

Chicken

Fish

Beef

Lamb

Pork

Salads and Veggies

Desserts

Testimonials

THE BIG CHANGE

The flames flew up from the fire melting the ice cream container I had in my hand. They rose up over my fingertips and down my palm and along the inside of my arm to my elbow. My satin shirt flapped in the light breeze as it too went up in flames.

My left side of my brain said, "Jump onto the ground and roll." The right side of my brain said, "No, the melting shirt will stick to your skin." The left side of my brain won, I rolled. It had been an incredibly silly thing to do throwing petrol onto a fire that I was trying to start.

I had recently become a single mother with four small children, the youngest only a month old. I quickly bundled them into my car. By the time I was at hospital some of the top layer of skin near my elbow had rubbed off.

In hospital they made me shower in cold water and injected me with morphine. It didn't seem to numb the pain at all. After a few hours my ex-husband arrived at the hospital and we were allowed to leave with my arm and stomach bandaged, (as they would not let me leave the hospital alone high on morphine).

For the next week alone with four small children (My ex could not stay). I would go to the local medical center, where a nurse would change my bandages and growl at me for putting Aloe vera leaves on my burns.

I would slice the leaf long ways down the middle and place the Aloe vera on my skin. The first time I put it on my skin it was the day after the fire, and sadly I wished I had put it on earlier as it soothed my still burning skin and relieved the pain.

The nurse treated me with Savlon cream on, and re-bandaging me, I would returned home and wash it off as my arm had started to swell and go red and hot. I would re-apply the Aloe vera. This soothed the redness and stopped the swelling. After three visits in that first week I stopped going to the nurse.

Where the skin had come off near my elbow and on my stomach an infection had set in. It was amazing to watch the infection come off onto the Aloe vera leaf when I would remove the older dry leaf to replace it with a fresh one at the beginning and end of each day.

I also found it really hard to keep the Aloe vera on my stomach as it would move around as I did. Being alone, I had to wash, clean, feed and look after the kids. All were between the ages of seven and new born.

My left hand looked like a blown up surgical glove with seams in it from all the lines on my hands. I had heard of Aloe vera being a great plant for burns and I was surprised at how quickly and well it healed my arm, and hand. Today it is hard to tell I was burnt as there is only minor discoloration to the area near my elbow where it was infected.

My stomach has a fair bit more scaring and discoloration, it was badly infected and it was harder to keep the Aloe vera over the scare as it kept moving as I did.

A few years later I heard about Aloe vera as a tonic to help people feel healthier.

I had two skin spots on my cheek and one on my bottom lip as I had been in the sun all my life, so I placed the Aloe vera on the sun spots and they went after about six months. My house sold and when we moved I only took a few mature Aloe vera plants with me.

After a few years I started to drink the Aloe vera juice again, about once a fortnight as I still didn't have many plants. I had started to get arthritis pain in my right hand and I was hoping it might relieve the pain.

The other skin cancer I still had on my bottom lip was like a scab that had been there now for at least seven years. I had taken my children and myself, to a mole specialist who spoke of some concerns about the scab on my lip. I later found it wasn't cancerous but it was a dangerous one that could grow extensively over the area causing serious damage to the tissues.

I drank the Aloe vera for six months to get rid of the arthritis. But found that it also got rid of my cold sores and eczema I have not had any of these things for over six years. Aloe vera only keeps it's potency for the first **two hours** after removing it from the plant. So it is better and very easy to **grow your own**.

On the 2nd of August 2008 my dog Maxine our eleven year old miniature foxy was diagnosed with liver cancer, she was bleeding from the bowel and could hardly walk. Her back legs were very weak and her balance was non existent. The Vet thought that she would only live for another week or two because she was so sick and small.

So I started to feed her Aloe vera and a crushed pain tablet which I would syringe into her mouth twice a day. After a month I noticed some benefit to her and she was still alive and very mentally alert. I decided to increase the Aloe vera intake to three times a day. After another three weeks her balance was remarkably better, and she was not bleeding from the bowel as much.

After twelve months all her arthritis was gone, we have now been arthritis free for over six years. Aloe vera is a herb, and it has 99% water and the one percent left has over 100 vitamins, minerals, enzymes and proteins in it making it a super food that we all need in our daily lives. Scientists and doctors have a research paper on Herbswisdom.com that explains all the vitamins and minerals and the 30 years of research they have done on this plant.

When you are healthy, drinking Aloe vera 1-2 times a week is sufficient. But when you are sick drinking and eating the Aloe vera three times a day is very important.

The medical Aloe vera has three main plants, the ***Candelabra*** is the strongest but it is a small vine type succulent, which the Asians like to use but after it has grown for at least seven years as it does not have much gel in it though. There is a yellow flowering plant, called the ***Barbadensis***, the orangey-red flowering plant is called ***Chinensis*** and is more commonly used in most gardens these two can be used after two years of growth. It is also **very important to eat healthy to stay healthy**, to **never neglect going to see your doctor** when you are sick, not just eat and drink this way, as it is **important to do both**.

When using a plant make sure that it is at least **two years old**, that you plant it in a sunny spot, or semi shade and it will grow well in a pot, but it will grow much better in a garden bed.

Dr Jill Rosemary Davies from the UK, has a degree in herbal medicine. She has also written a book called "In a nutshell Aloe vera." Her book also talks of the great healing properties of this plant and if taken smartly with healthy food we can teach our bodies to heal a lot of illnesses and diseases. Her book can be found in most libraries throughout the world.

Dr Davies also talks about how her research has found that the Egyptians used Aloe vera five thousand years ago and that in the nineteenth century the Aloe vera was dropped by many and only used for a few ailments.

> *"Aloe vera can treat so many more ailments than first discovered. If we continue researching who knows where it could lead. Each and every day my research brings new and wonderful findings from this plant,"* says Dr Jill Davies.

Note: When using a leaf, make sure it is at least two years old, and around six to eight inches in length. Always make sure you wash the leaf before using it as it has a yellow sap that is quite bitter and can cause a laxative effect or a rash. This is it's natural protectant against insects and animals attacking it and it only occurs in the first cut.

Dr. Simoncini came out with some new findings about cancer and the **University of California Irvine Researchers** team also came out with the same findings. That we have fungus, bacteria and cancer cells in our bodies all the time but our immune system while strong and healthy keeps them in small amounts. So when the immune system gets low these things grow to much larger levels. Making it vitally important we keep our immune system healthy. Aloe vera is a great natural way of doing that, and when you grow your own it is also very cost effective.

FIRST STEPS TO GROWING & USING ALOE VERA

(fresh is always better)

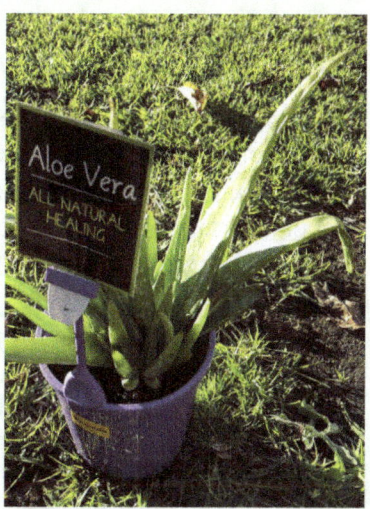

Where to find plants:
- Your local gardening nursery
- An Aloe vera farm
- From a friend or neighbour who has some plants already
- At a garage sale

Look for the *barbadensis* and *chinensis* varieties which are the best for health use. Please observe local laws, i.e. avoid taking wild-growing plants out of natural environments.

How to care for your plants:
- Aloe vera plants dislike being crowded. Separate each plant into its own pot. Select a pot with good drainage that is large enough to fit the size of an adult plant. If planting in a veggie patch, keep the plants at least 60cm (2 feet) apart.
- Aloe vera is hardy and can go weeks without water. However, it is advised to water your plants daily to maintain optimal strong growth.
- Experiment with positioning to ensure your plants get suitable amounts of sunlight, around 6 to 8 hours a day. If the leaves turn yellow in colour, move them to a spot with more shade.

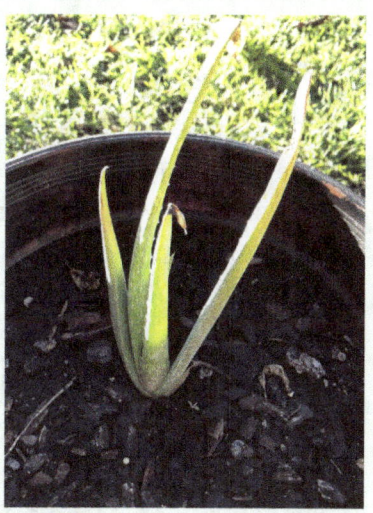

When the leaves are ready to use:
- It takes a year or two to develop a mature leaf that is high in goodness.
- Always use mature leaves that are at least 23cm (7 inches) long. A good marker is to only use leaves that are growing below where the most recent flower-stalk grew.
- It is always better to cut the leaf with a sharp knife because just snapping the leaf off can cause stress and damage to the plant.
- Wash thoroughly and rinse off the yellow sap as it is tastes bitter and may cause a mild rash or mild laxative effect if ingested.
- The goodness in processed gel lasts for about two hours and whole leaves for about a day in the fridge. A great way to preserve it is to blend the gel with water, fill ice cube trays, then just pop it in the freezer.
- If you are using it on your scalp or body, just cut off the size you need rather than an entire leaf to avoid wastage.

HERBS AND THEIR IMPRESSIVE USE

In a recent article in the Medical Journal of Australia and accompanying position paper from the US. Claims of culinary herbs and spices containing high concentrations of antioxidants and photo nutrients provide long term health benefits which far outweigh the short term taste sensations you get when using them.

The antioxidants identified include *anthocyanins*, *flavonoids*, *phenolic acids*, *sulphur* – containing compounds and *monoterpenes*. They are also very rich in vitamins, minerals and other bioactive components. Other studies show they act synergistically to enhance the health related properties of other foods **and to multiply their antioxidant value in a meal.**

So when using herbs, fresh is best! They are great when combined with different foods not just for flavor but also for their health value. Aloe vera being the strongest from the herb family is highly recommended.

It is wonderful to see the medical profession is recognizing the qualities of herbs and the importance of having them in our daily meals with fresh raw veggies and fruits in salads.

> An informative herbal book is called HOW CAN I USE HERBS IN MY DAILY LIFE. It is written by Isabell Shipard and you can find out more information by contacting her through her website on http://www.herbsarespecial.com.au.

GROWING ALOE VERA IS EASY

Aloe vera barbadensis. F Asphodelaceae.

When you buy an Aloe vera plant, try to ask for one that's around two years old so you can use it immediately. You might pay less for a younger plant that hasn't had a chance to grow flowers yet. For eating uses, Aloe vera plants need time to grow and mature properly so that the gel has over 100 vitamins and minerals in it that we need.

When purchasing for the first time, be aware that there are several varieties of Aloe vera plants. Know what the Barbadensis and chinensis aloe vera looks like by googling Aloe vera images.

If you are planting in the garden, give your plants a warm sunny spot that gets some shade. Aloe vera are originally from Africa, so they love the sun, and don't like temperatures below ten degrees Celsius.

So if you are in a cool climate, plant it in a pot and keep it in a warm green-house, or inside will be fine, in the cooler months. Make sure there's plenty of growing room in the pot.

In the warm Australian weather, here in South East Queensland, my plants are outside all year round. I water them regularly and make sure the soil is not too dry. I like to keep the saucer under the plant pot full of water.

The Aloe vera, like most cacti, grows babies - also known as pups. When you have several pups you can gently prize them from the adult plant without removing the adult. If they are in a pot then it is best to remove all of the little plants from the pot, and also refresh the soil anyway. The plant does not grow big with too many in the same pot and the bigger the plant the more vitamins and minerals it will have. So try to keep it to one plant per pot.

They love a sandy soil that dries out fairly quickly. In the garden, they can soon grow into thick clusters of many plants if looked after well. When friends come around, you can pluck a plant from below, trying to keep some roots on the stalk, to give and let them grow in their own garden.

When you want to cut off a leaf to use it, you must remember to **use it within the first two hours of cutting it** as most of the goodness dies after two hours. If you put all the cutting and waste of the leaf back into the soil it will self compost and help the plant to be really healthy. Also if you rinse the yellow sap off in a bowl of water you can then put the sap water into a water spray bottle and use that on your veggies and herbs to prevent other animals and insects from attacking it.

DISCLAIMER

Always consult a qualified and licensed medical specialist
when trying any new changes to your usual eating habits.

© Copyright 2010-2019

"Cookin' for Cures"
by Angie Andrews

Typeset by phormulae.com

First Edition eBook released in June 2010 and updated in October 2010.
Second Edition eBook released in May 2012.
Third Edition eBook released September 2013.
Fourth Edition eBook released December 2014.
This (Fifth) Edition eBook released July 2019.
This (Fifth) Edition hardcopy also released in 2019.
(Angie's Smart Books ISBN 978-064654587-5)

Hardcopy released in November 2012.
(Joshua Books ISBN 978-098718489-4)

Please consult the author for express permission before using the materials
in this e-book for any kind of financially beneficial derivative works.

Please visit, www.angiessmartbooks.com

DRINK FOR GOOD HEALTH

Fruit and veggies are very popular in drinks and can be easy to make. Use all the variety of fruits and veggies you like, even the ones you don't! They can be masked with fruit to level out the flavour.

Nutritionists claim that the majority of the goodness is in the fiber or pulp, it is still of great benefit to have a fresh juice every morning. It would be far more beneficial than having a coffee with breakfast. If you must, you can have both though.

Some of the remaining pulp can be added into a pancake or omelet mix if you are making them for breakfast that morning. As it is important to remember that it must be eaten straight away to get the best benefits from the Aloe vera.

When my dog's symptoms worsened, it confirmed the fact that the Aloe vera had lost most of its healing qualities. It had been in the fridge for half a day.

The more raw fruit and veggies we have in our meals the healthier we will be, with the addition of Aloe vera, we should not only live healthier but longer lives.

If you incorporate only one or two of these recipes in your daily meals you will feel the benefits. **Always ensure that you rinse the Aloe vera leaf thoroughly to remove the yellow sap from the leaf. The yellow aloe latex is bitter, and can cause a rash or the runs when ingested.**

Aloe vera is Amazing!

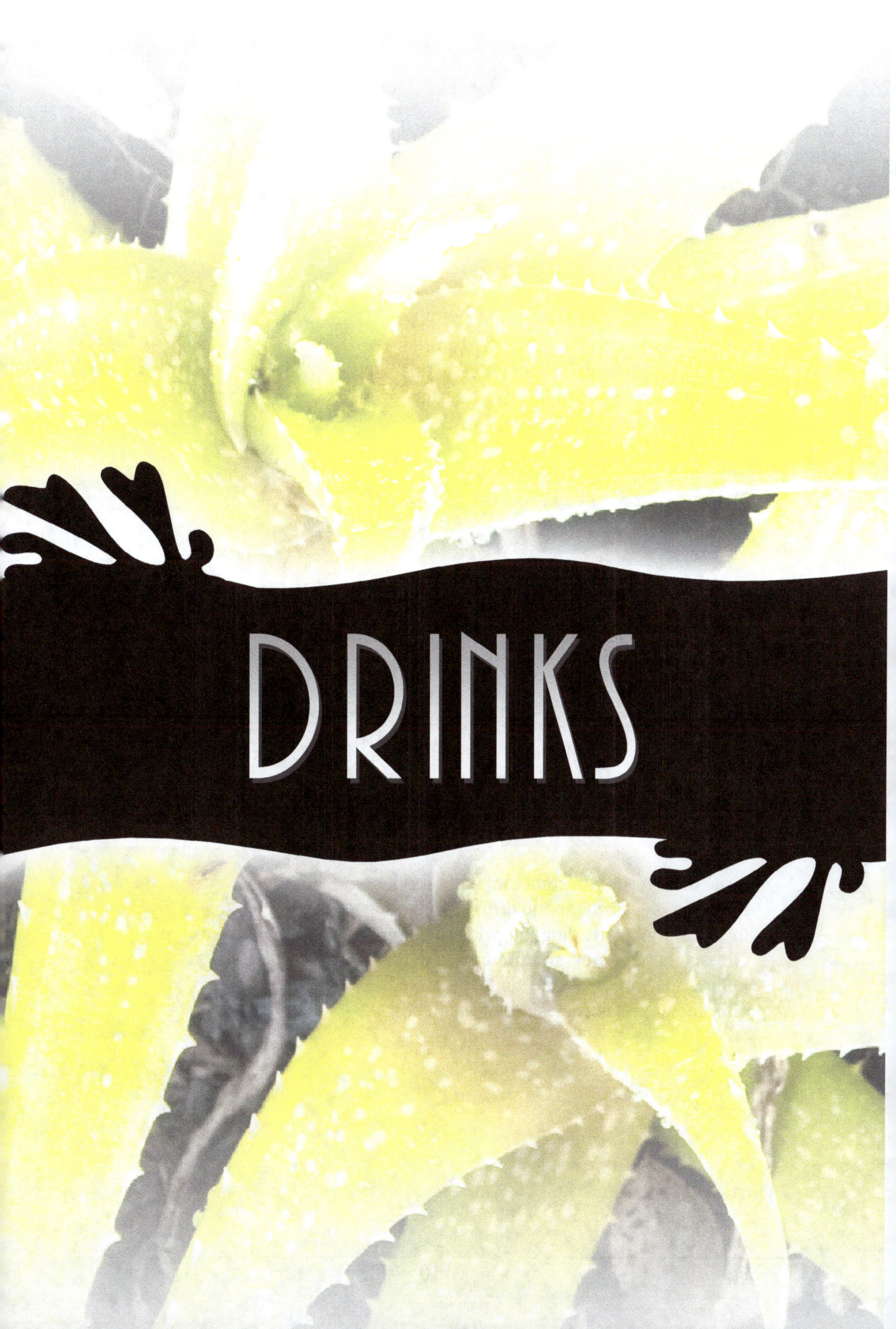

ALOE VERA JUICE
(regenerate cells)

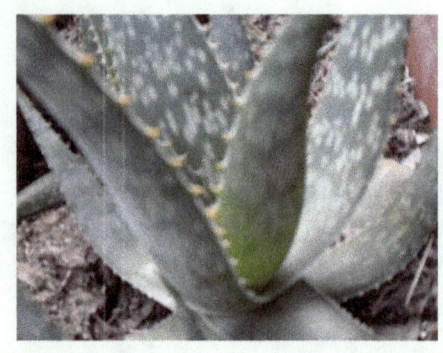

Ingredients:
2 Aloe vera leaves

1) Rinse the leaf thoroughly first to remove the yellow stain from the leaf as this has a bitter taste and can cause the runs or a rash on the skin.

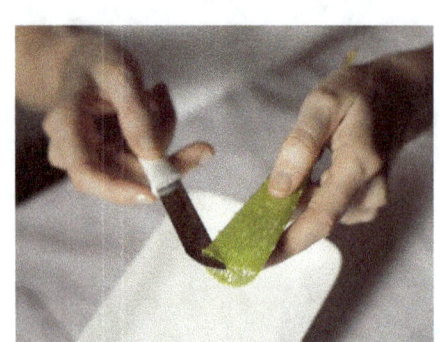

2) Cut two, six to eight inch long leaves of Aloe vera.

3) Trim sides to remove the prickles, (I use scissors) with a sharp knife slice down the center of the leaf of the leaf from the side to reveal the gel.

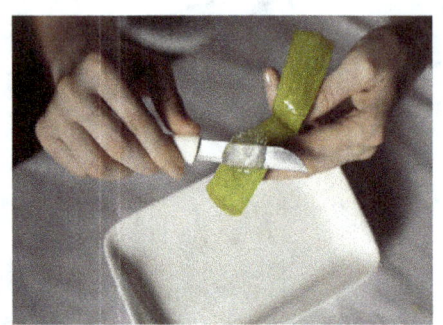

4) Scrape all the gel into a jug and use an electric blender to mix the gel down into a liquid.

It is then ready to combine with food or juice. To make a smoothie drink, simply add the juice to the blending jug prior to mixing. Aloe vera will not go through a juicer / juicing machine, so it needs to be mixed in after the juice has comes out of the juicer.

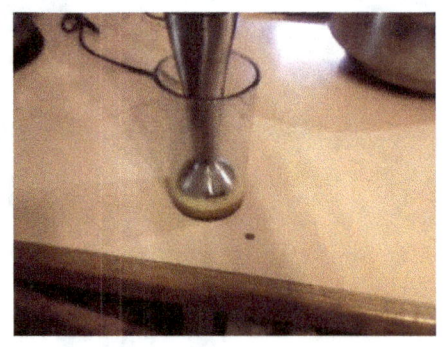

Cookin' for Cures

ALOE POWER DRINK
(keeps you hydrated and helps you recover from gastro)

Ingredients
1 Aloe vera leaf
1 cup of Powerade

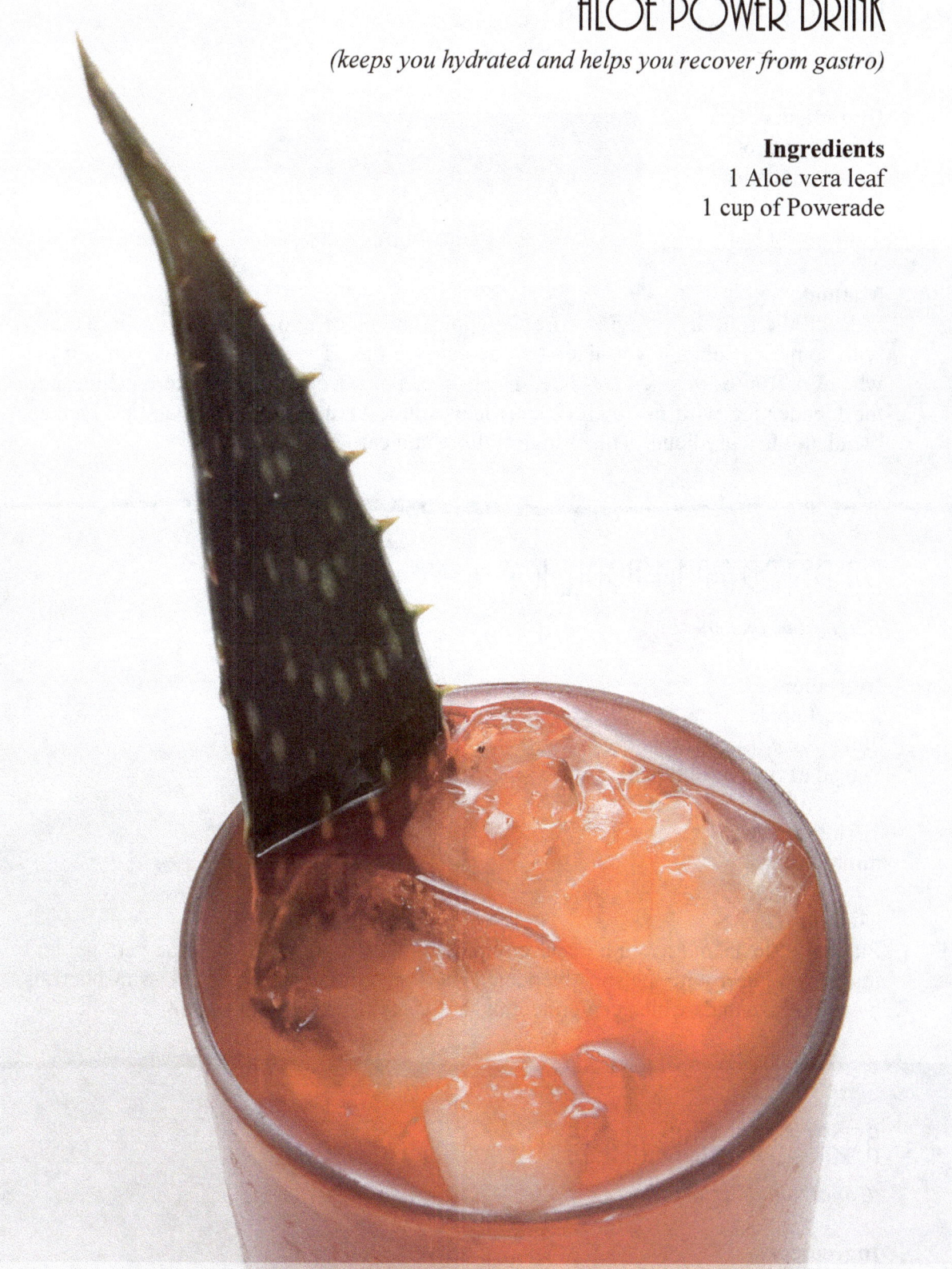

Method
Put Aloe vera into blender jug add Powerade and blend together and add ice.

APPLE AND CARROT JUICE

(Energy Drink)

Ingredients
1 medium apple
1 medium carrot
1 handful of beans
1 Aloe vera leaf

Method
Slice all the fruit and veggies, core the apple, and place into a juicer. Pour into a cup with some ice cubes if you like. As you can see this is very simple and you can put whatever fruit or veggies you like. Then place the juice from the juice machine into the blender jug with 6-8 inch (20cm) leaves aloe vera gel and with a stick blender blend all the ingredients. This is high in fibre and carotene.

RASPBERRY AND APPLE ICY

(High fibre and energy)

Ingredients
2 sweet apples
200g (7oz / 0.4lb) raspberries
¼ tspn of Stevia (optional)
4 cups of ice
1 Aloe vera leaf
mint for garnish

Method
Put fruit, Stevia and ice in a juicer and process until smooth. Blend aloe vera gel and juice from juicer with the stick blender. This is a great anti-cancer drink as raspberries have bioflavonoids which can protect the body against cancer formation.

ASPARAGUS AND APPLE

(Cancer inhibiter drink)

Ingredients
1 hand full of fresh asparagus
2 apples
1 Aloe vera leaf

Method
Combine the apple and asparagus into a juicer with ice, then add to the aloe, blend with the blender, and serve immediately. The asparagus and aloe vera are very good at fighting off cancer cells, and the apples are great for fibre, also a good sweetener.

Asparagus and Apple

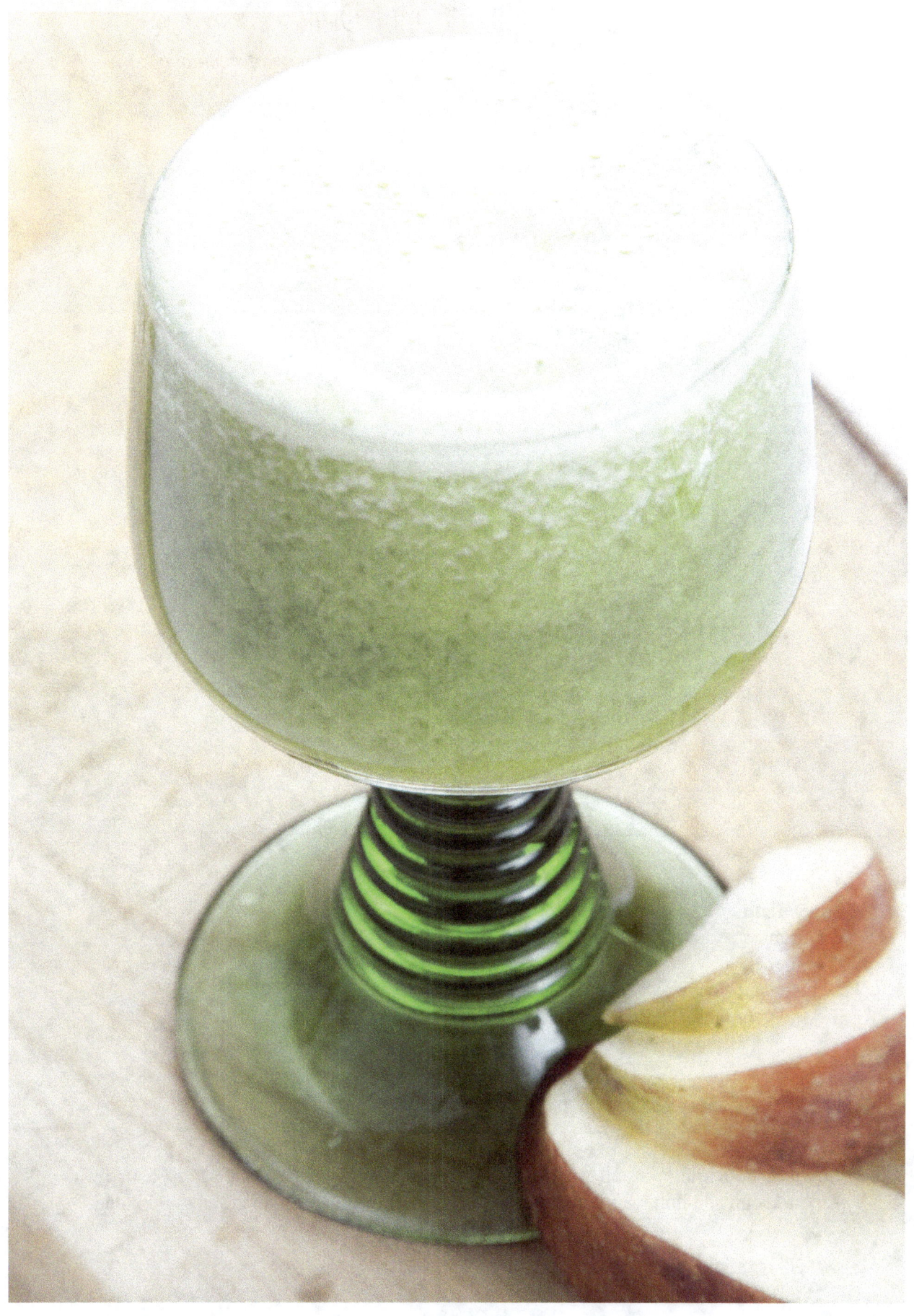

LEMON AND HONEY DRINK
(Colds and flu reducer, especially at the very beginning of symptoms)

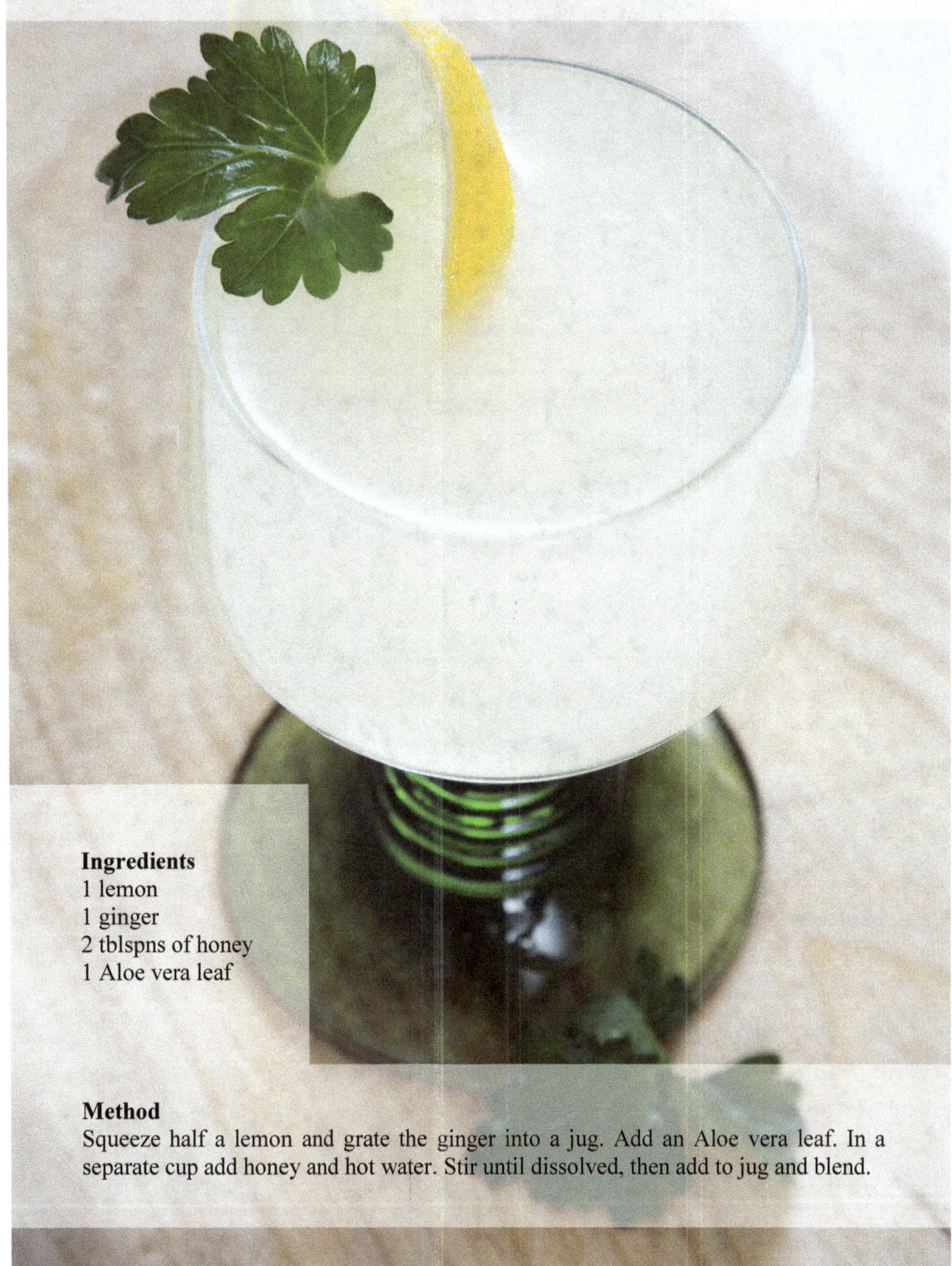

Ingredients
1 lemon
1 ginger
2 tblspns of honey
1 Aloe vera leaf

Method
Squeeze half a lemon and grate the ginger into a jug. Add an Aloe vera leaf. In a separate cup add honey and hot water. Stir until dissolved, then add to jug and blend.

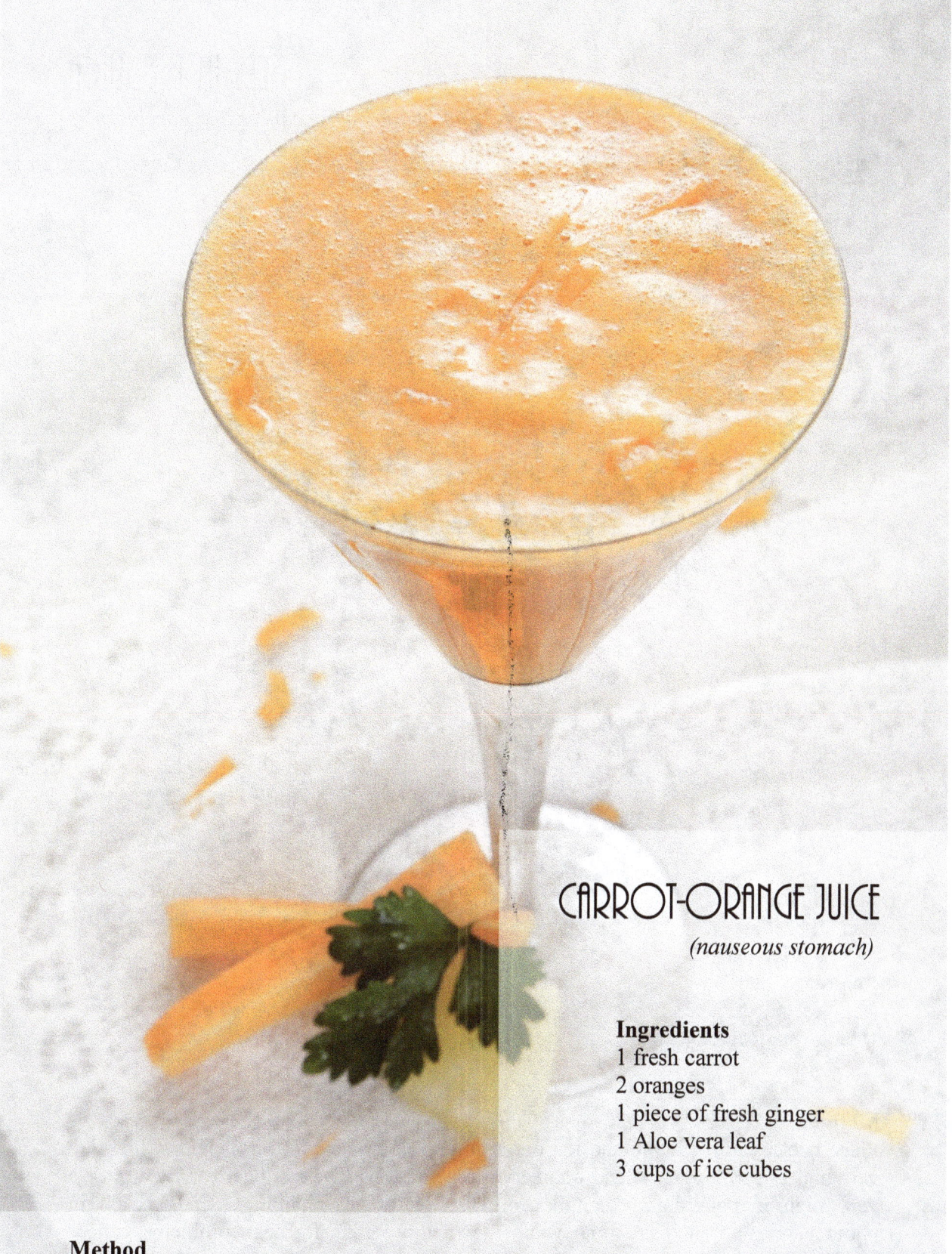

CARROT-ORANGE JUICE
(nauseous stomach)

Ingredients
1 fresh carrot
2 oranges
1 piece of fresh ginger
1 Aloe vera leaf
3 cups of ice cubes

Method
Place carrots and oranges into a juicer. Pour juice into a blender with Aloe vera and grated ginger. Blend. This is a great one to have when you are not feeling the best. Fresh ginger is very good at getting rid of stomach upsets.

BEET IN THE JUICE
(great for heart disease cancer and Parkinson's)

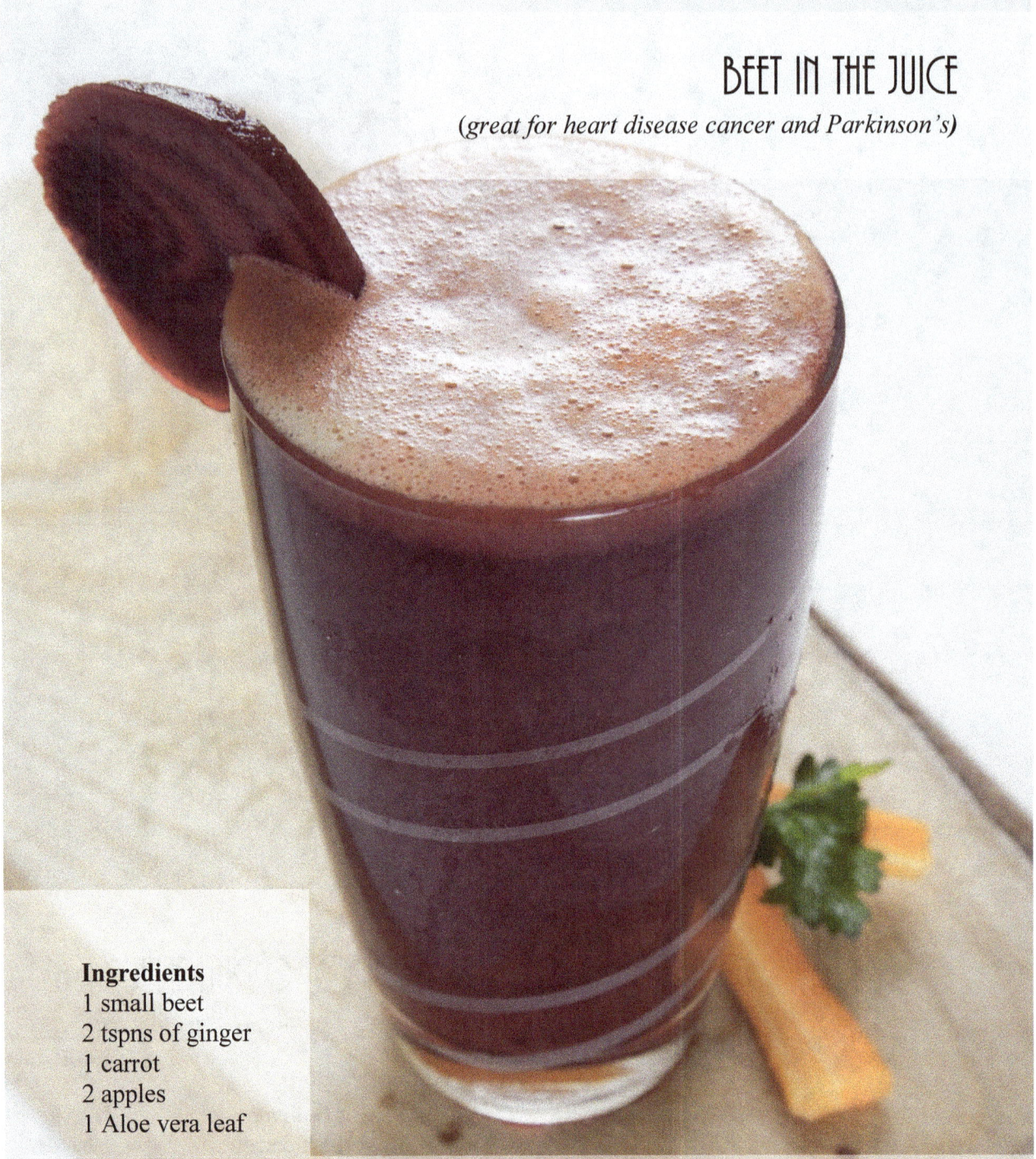

Ingredients
1 small beet
2 tspns of ginger
1 carrot
2 apples
1 Aloe vera leaf

Method
Place beets, carrots, apple and ice into a juicer. Pour juice into a blender with Aloe vera and grated ginger. Blend and serve immediately. The red beet (or Beetroot) is very high in potassium, calcium, iron, beta carotene, vitamin C and is rich in photochemicals - such as Anthocyanins - which are great for heart problems, cancer and Parkinson's disease.

Important Note: The dye in the red beet can turn the urine and stools red so don't get worried and think you are bleeding.

FRUITY VEGGIE DRINK
(for the heart)

Ingredients
1 carrot
1 stalk of celery
1 apple
1 mandarin
1 Aloe vera leaf

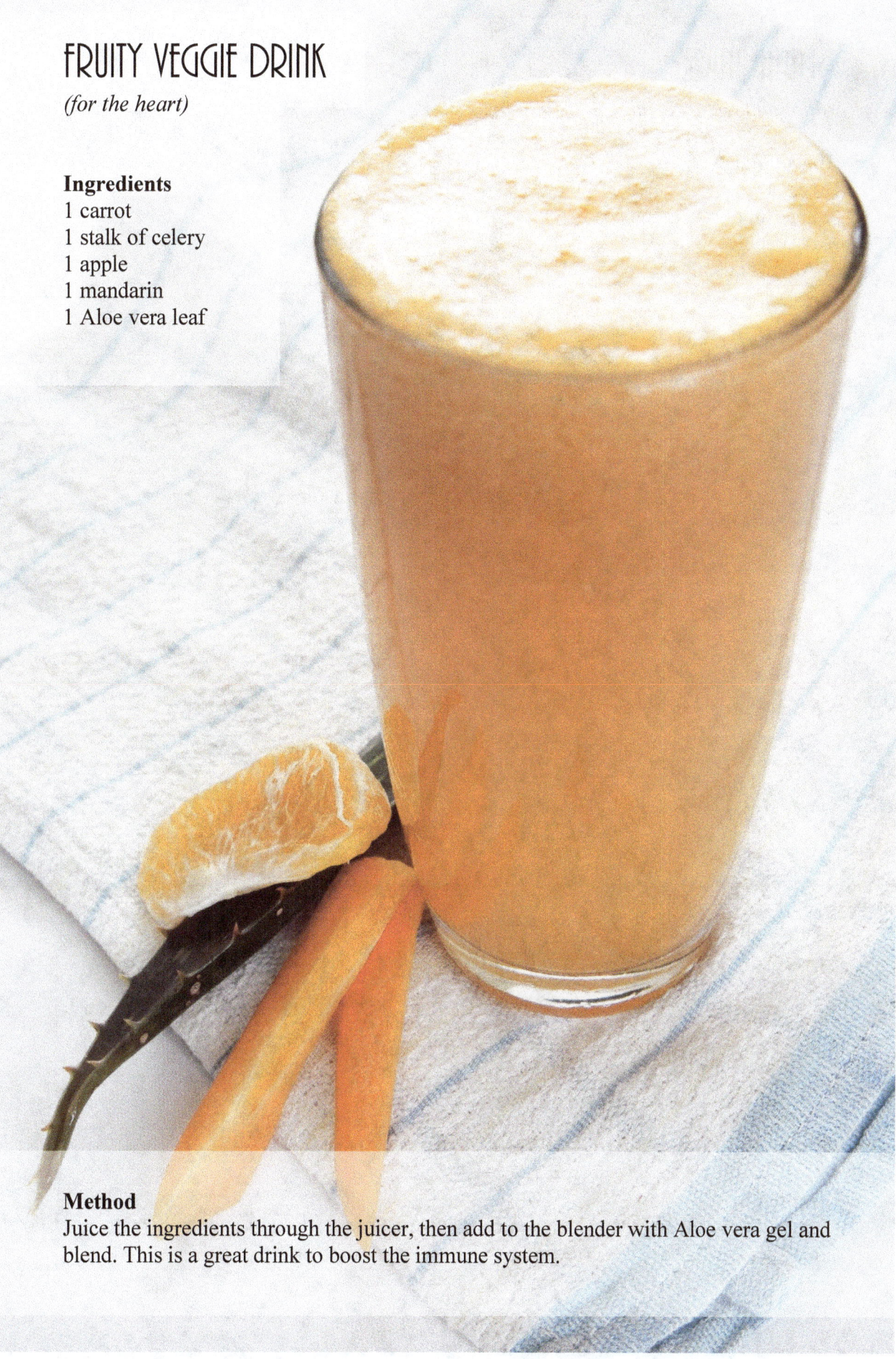

Method
Juice the ingredients through the juicer, then add to the blender with Aloe vera gel and blend. This is a great drink to boost the immune system.

BEANIE JUICE
(fibre and energy drink)

Ingredients
1 carrot
1 handful of raw green beans
2 or 3 apples to taste
1 Aloe vera leaf

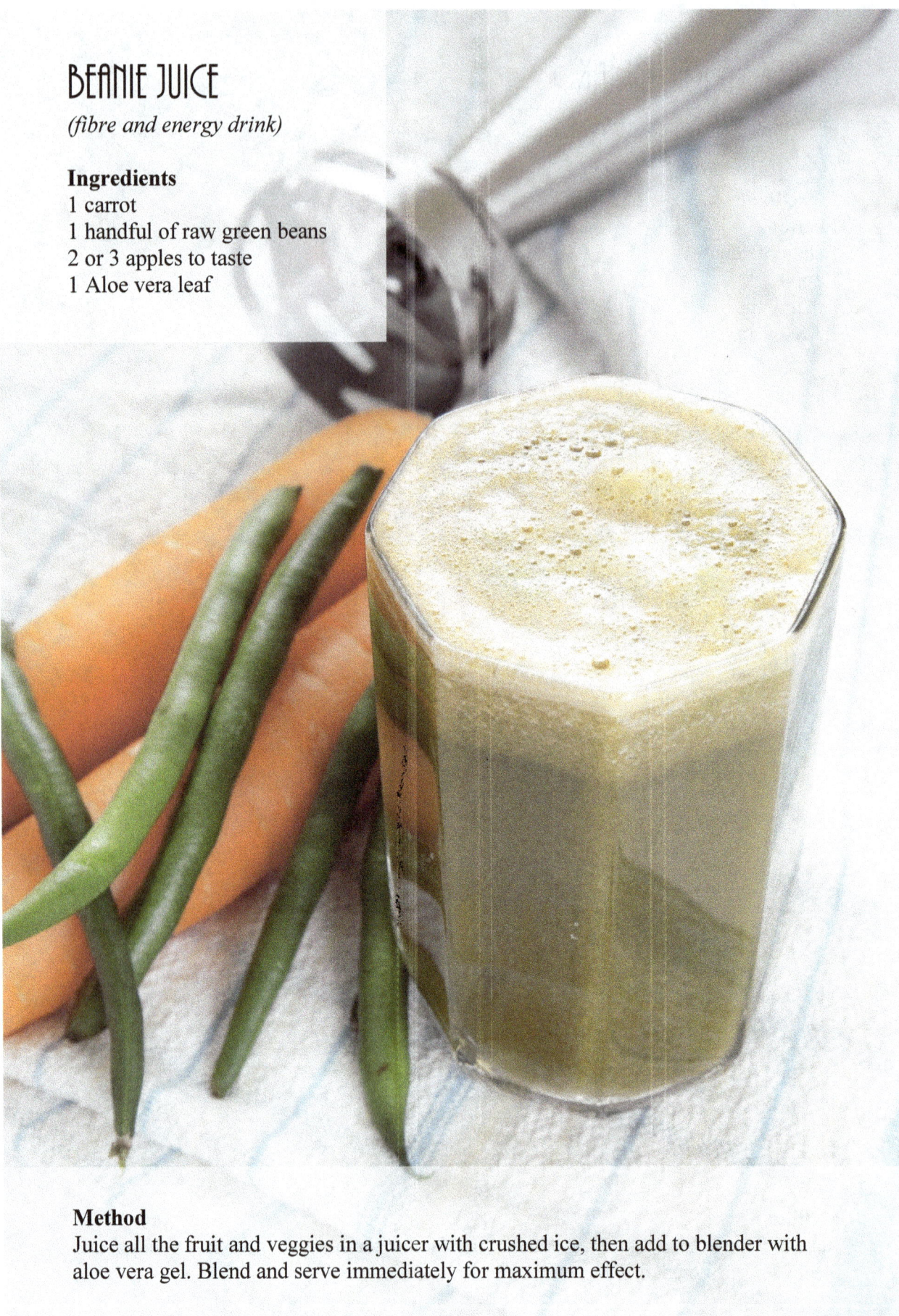

Method
Juice all the fruit and veggies in a juicer with crushed ice, then add to blender with aloe vera gel. Blend and serve immediately for maximum effect.

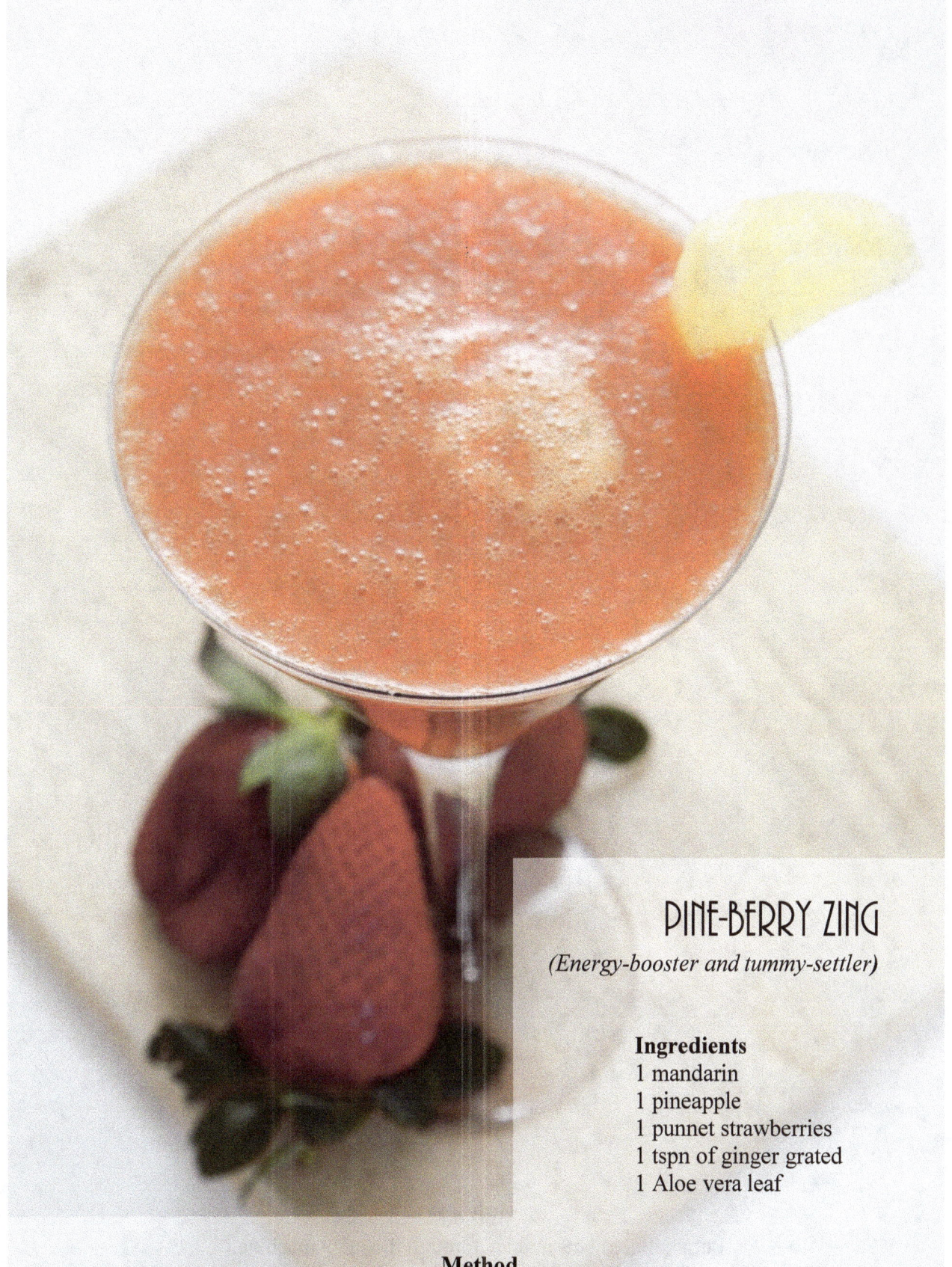

PINE-BERRY ZING
(Energy-booster and tummy-settler)

Ingredients
1 mandarin
1 pineapple
1 punnet strawberries
1 tspn of ginger grated
1 Aloe vera leaf

Method
Juice all the fruit and veggies in a juicer with crushed ice, then add to blender with aloe vera gel. Blend and serve.

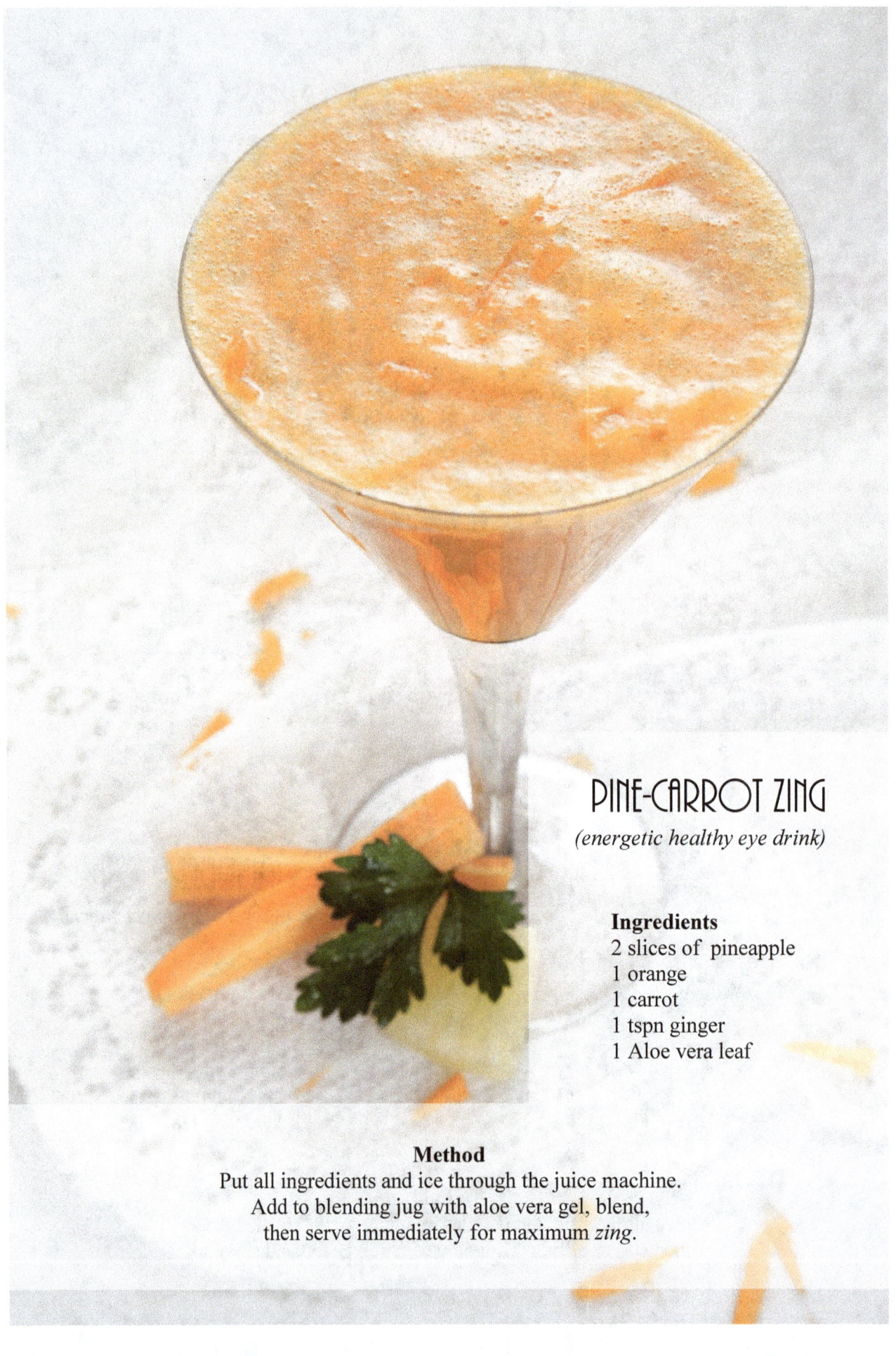

PINE-CARROT ZING
(energetic healthy eye drink)

Ingredients
2 slices of pineapple
1 orange
1 carrot
1 tspn ginger
1 Aloe vera leaf

Method
Put all ingredients and ice through the juice machine.
Add to blending jug with aloe vera gel, blend,
then serve immediately for maximum *zing*.

HAPPY MANGO JUICE
(sweet and regular)

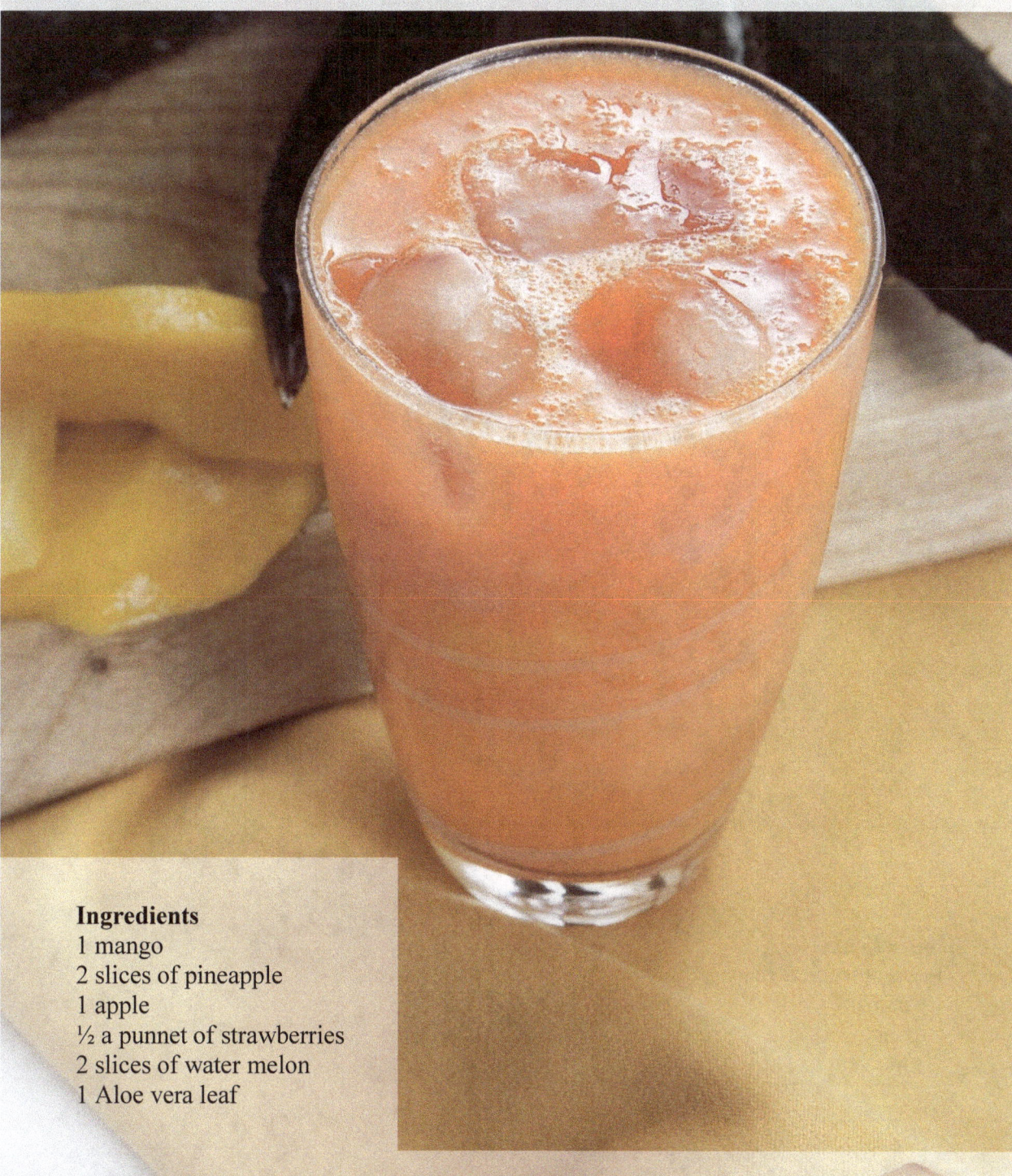

Ingredients
1 mango
2 slices of pineapple
1 apple
½ a punnet of strawberries
2 slices of water melon
1 Aloe vera leaf

Method
Put all ingredients and some ice through the juice machine, then add to blending jug with Aloe vera gel, blend and then serve. Mango and Pineapple are full of good fibre.

TROPICAL BLENDED JUICE
(high in Vitamin B C E and lots of fibre great for energy)

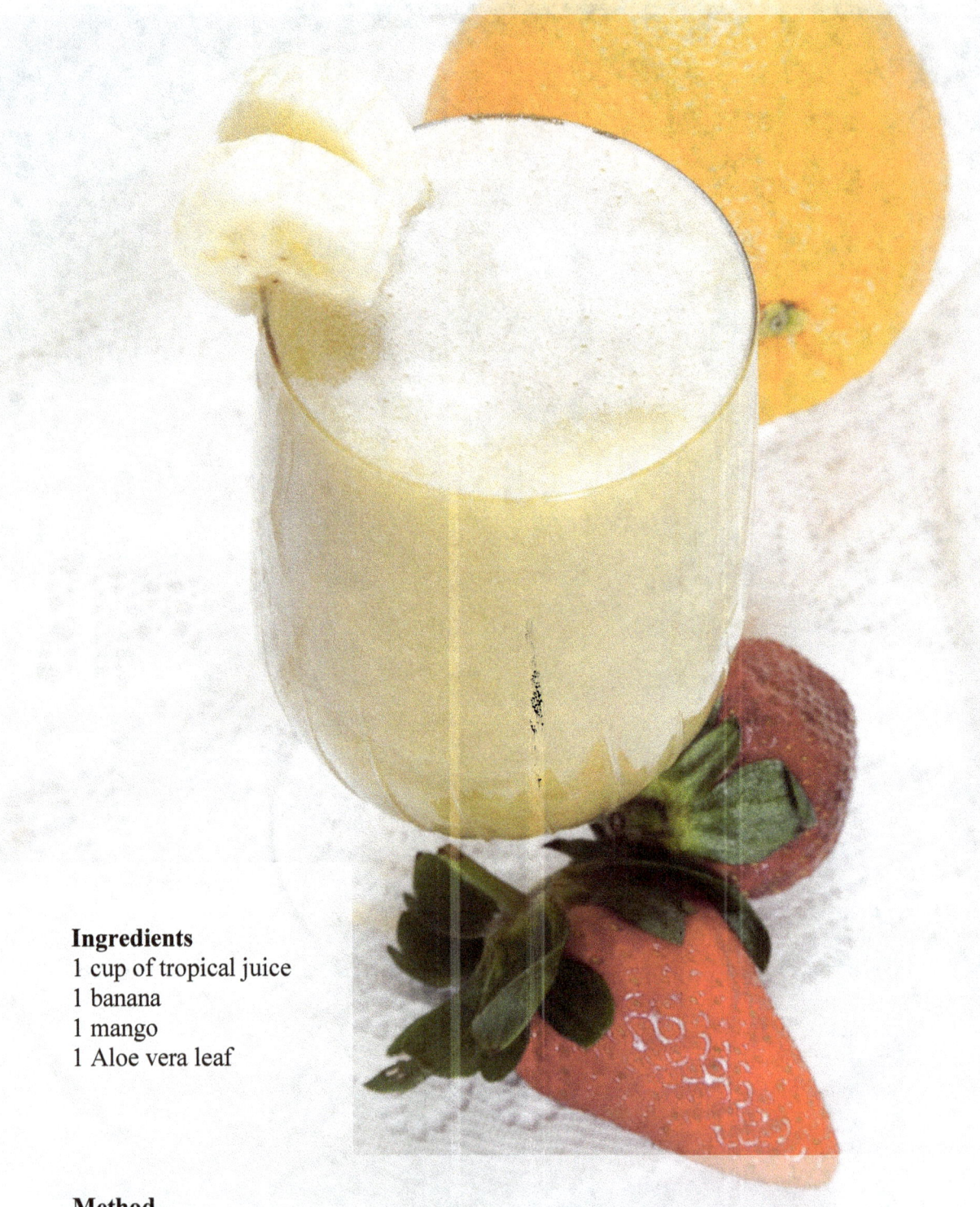

Ingredients
1 cup of tropical juice
1 banana
1 mango
1 Aloe vera leaf

Method
Put all ingredients and ice through the juice machine. Add to blender jug with Aloe vera gel, blend and then serve.

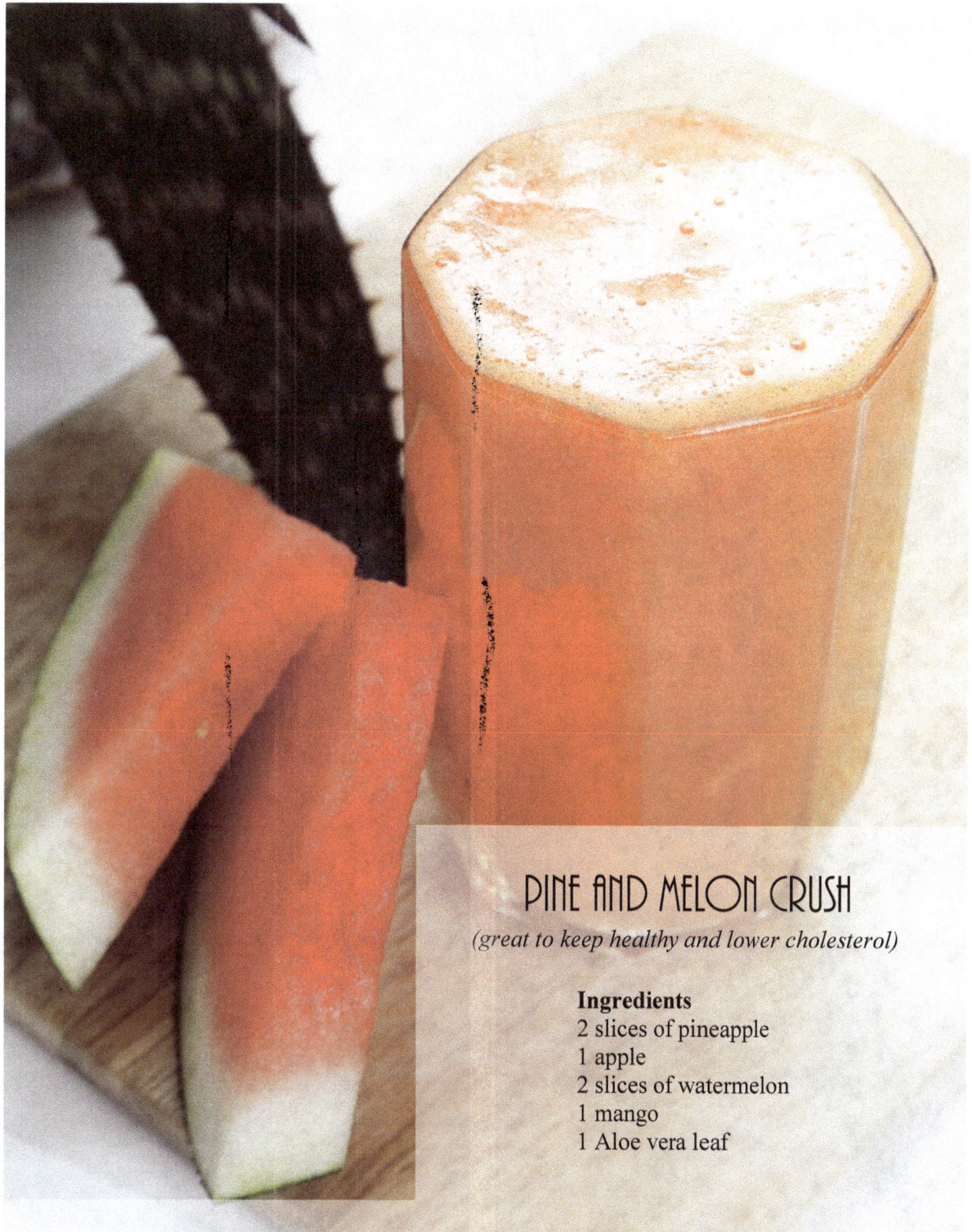

PINE AND MELON CRUSH
(great to keep healthy and lower cholesterol)

Ingredients
2 slices of pineapple
1 apple
2 slices of watermelon
1 mango
1 Aloe vera leaf

Method
Put all ingredients and ice through the juice machine,
add to blending jug with Aloe vera gel, blend and then serve.

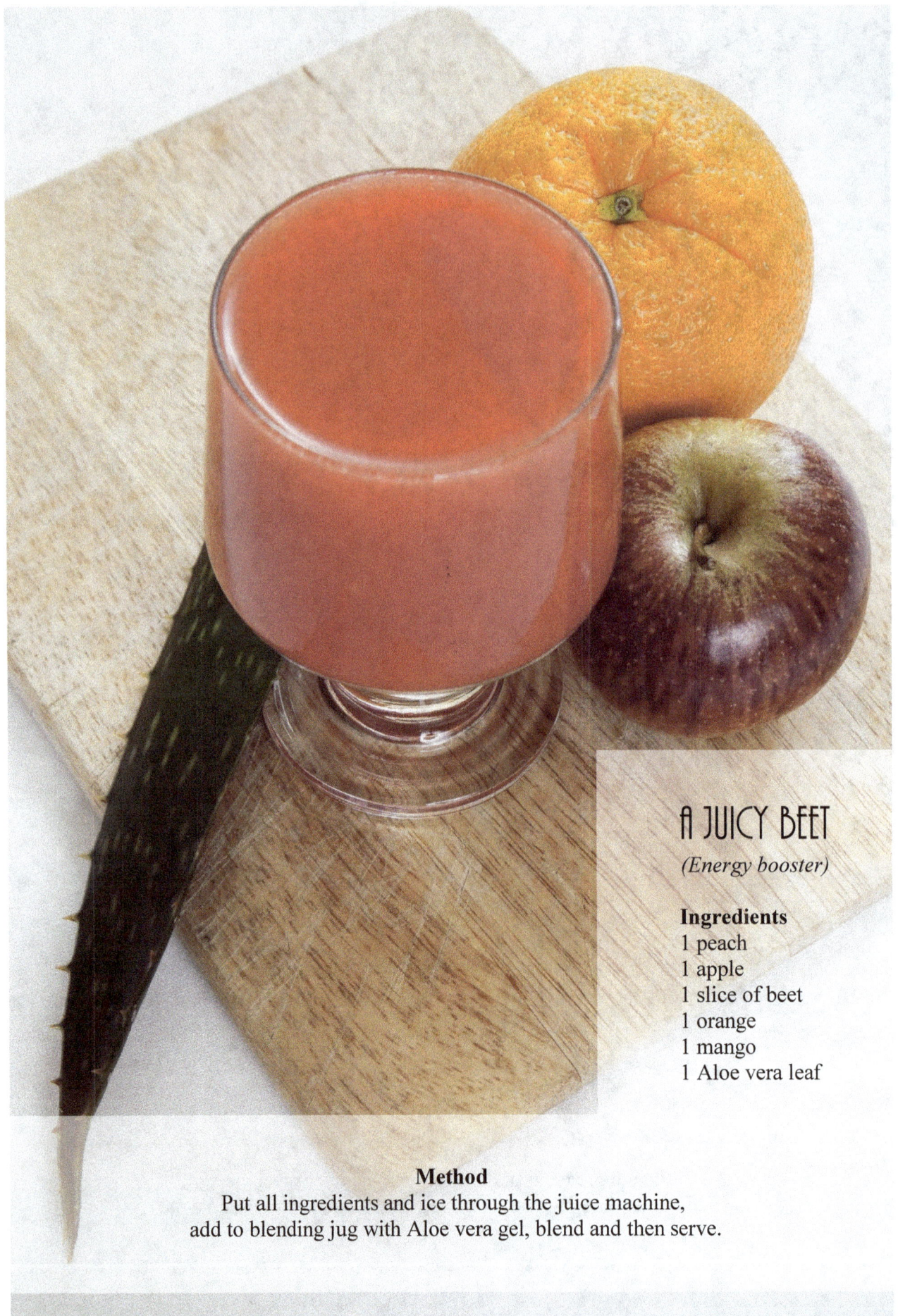

A JUICY BEET

(Energy booster)

Ingredients
1 peach
1 apple
1 slice of beet
1 orange
1 mango
1 Aloe vera leaf

Method
Put all ingredients and ice through the juice machine,
add to blending jug with Aloe vera gel, blend and then serve.

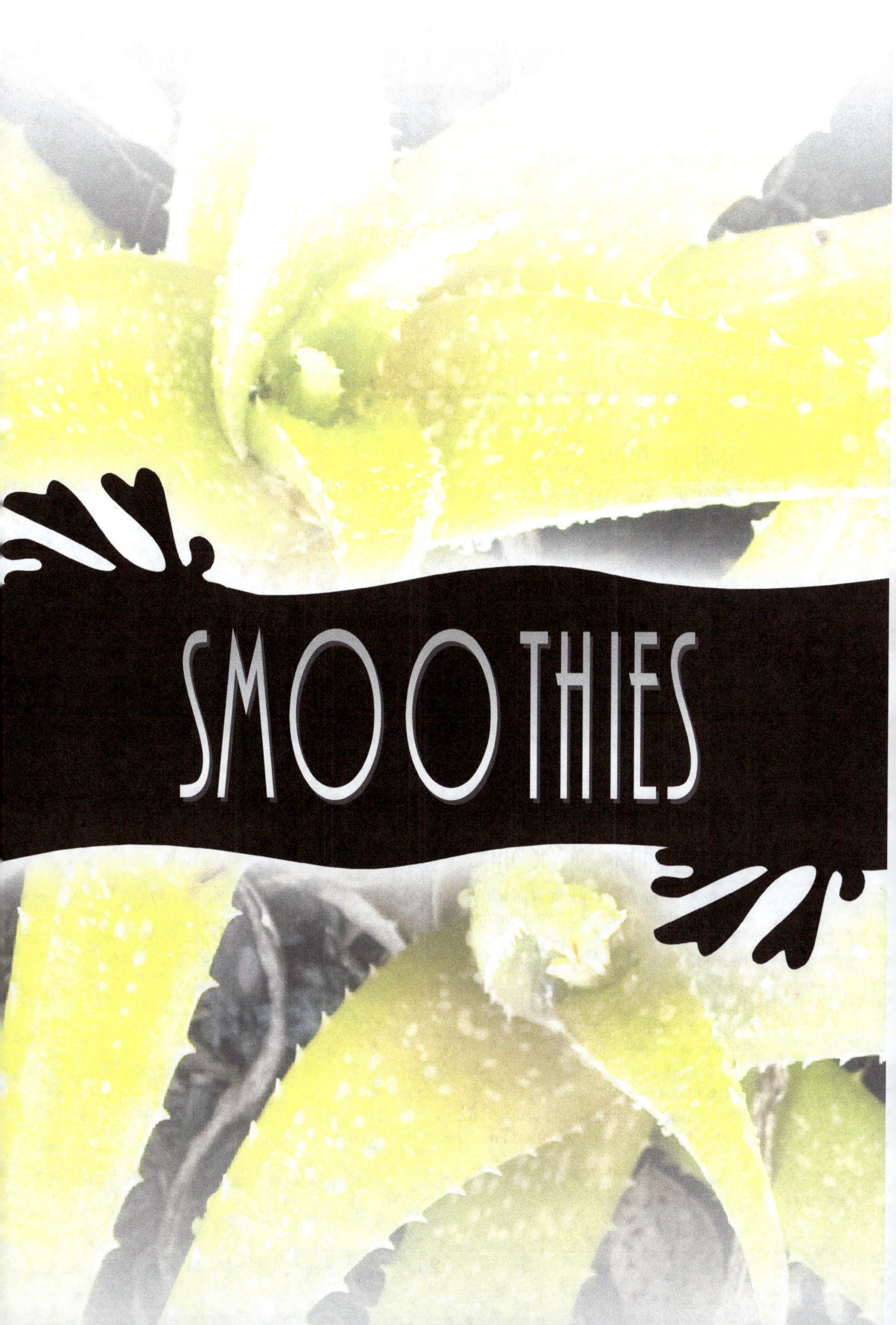

BAN-MANGO SMOOTHIE

(High B C and E helps remove body fats)

Ingredients
1 banana
1 mango
1 cup of vanilla yoghurt
1 Aloe vera leaf

Method
Juice banana, mango and crushed ice.
Add to blender jug with yoghurt and Aloe vera gel. Blend and serve.

PEACH ON THE GO

(Great for stomach ulcers and energy)

Ingredients
1 banana
1 mango
1 peach
1 cup of vanilla yoghurt
1 Aloe vera leaf

Method
Juice banana, mango, peach and crushed ice.
Add to blender jug with yoghurt and Aloe vera gel. Blend and serve.

PINE-ORANGE SMOOTHIE

(Vitamin C, high in fibre, and pineapple contains bromeliad enzymes which can help reduce the pain and swelling of arthritis)

Ingredients
2 slices of pineapple
1 orange
1 cup of vanilla yoghurt
1 Aloe vera leaf

Method
Juice pineapple, orange and crushed ice.
Add to blender jug with yoghurt and Aloe vera gel. Blend and serve.

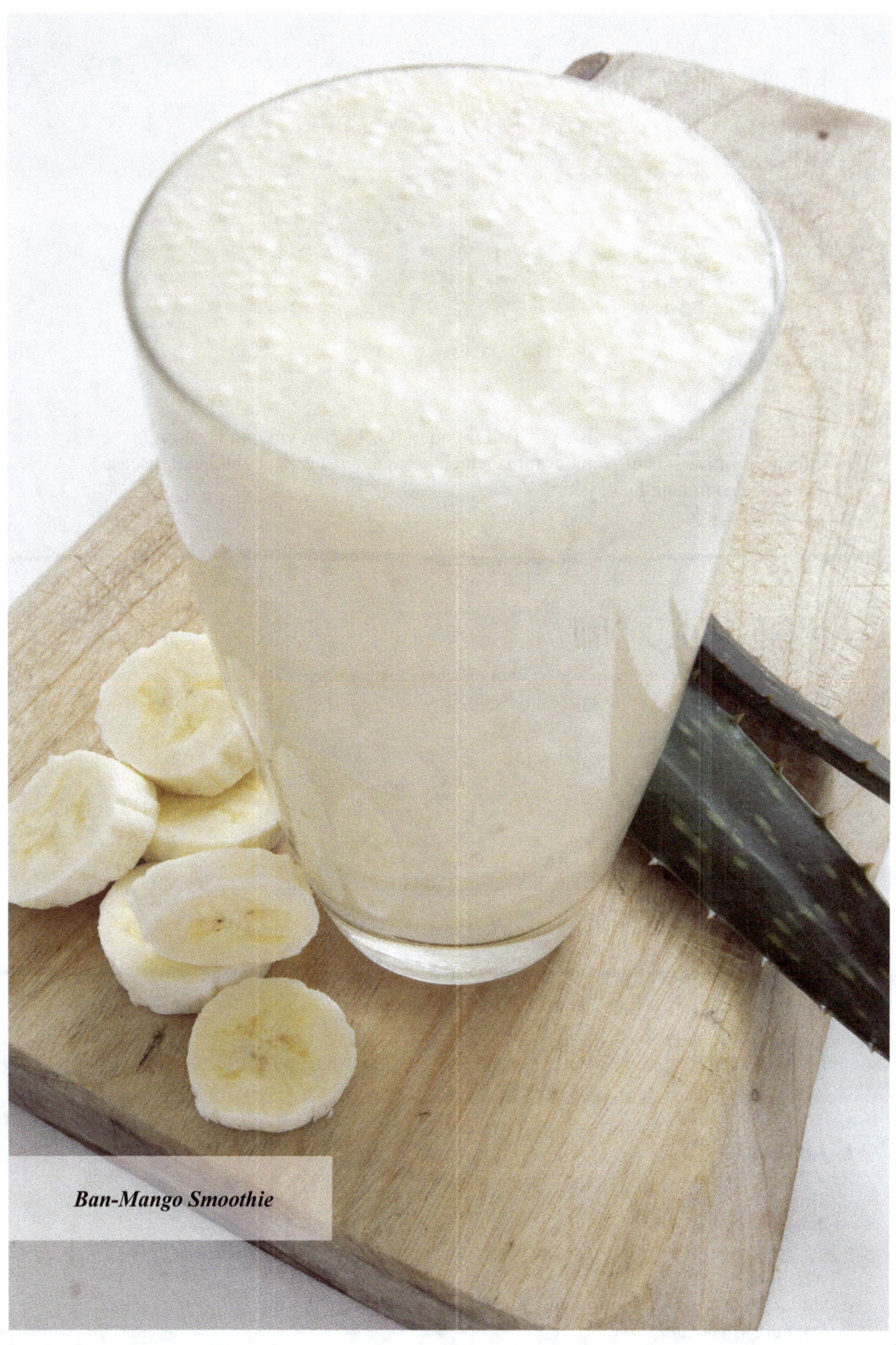
Ban-Mango Smoothie

BERRY SMOOTHIE

(fights against heart disease, cancer and Parkinson's)

Ingredients
1 cup yoghurt
1 punnet of strawberries
1 punnet of raspberries
1 punnet blue berries
1 Aloe vera leaf
crushed ice

Method
Blend all ingredients. This is a great all rounder, it is high in vitamin C, stops urine infections, it has lots of Anthocyanins which helps against cancer and heart disease. There is also iron and potassium.

APPLE AL SMOOTHIE

(energy, fibre and photochemicals that can help prevent heart disease)

Ingredients
2 apples
1 Aloe vera leaf
1 cup of vanilla yoghurt

Method
Put apple and crushed ice through a juicer. Add to blending jug with Aloe vera gel and yoghurt. Blend and serve.

MANDY AL SMOOTHIE

(high in vitamin C, beta carotene and potassium)

Ingredients
2 mandarins
1 apple
1 Aloe vera leaf

Method
Put apple and mandarin through a juicer. Add to blending jug with Aloe vera gel and yoghurt. Blend and serve.

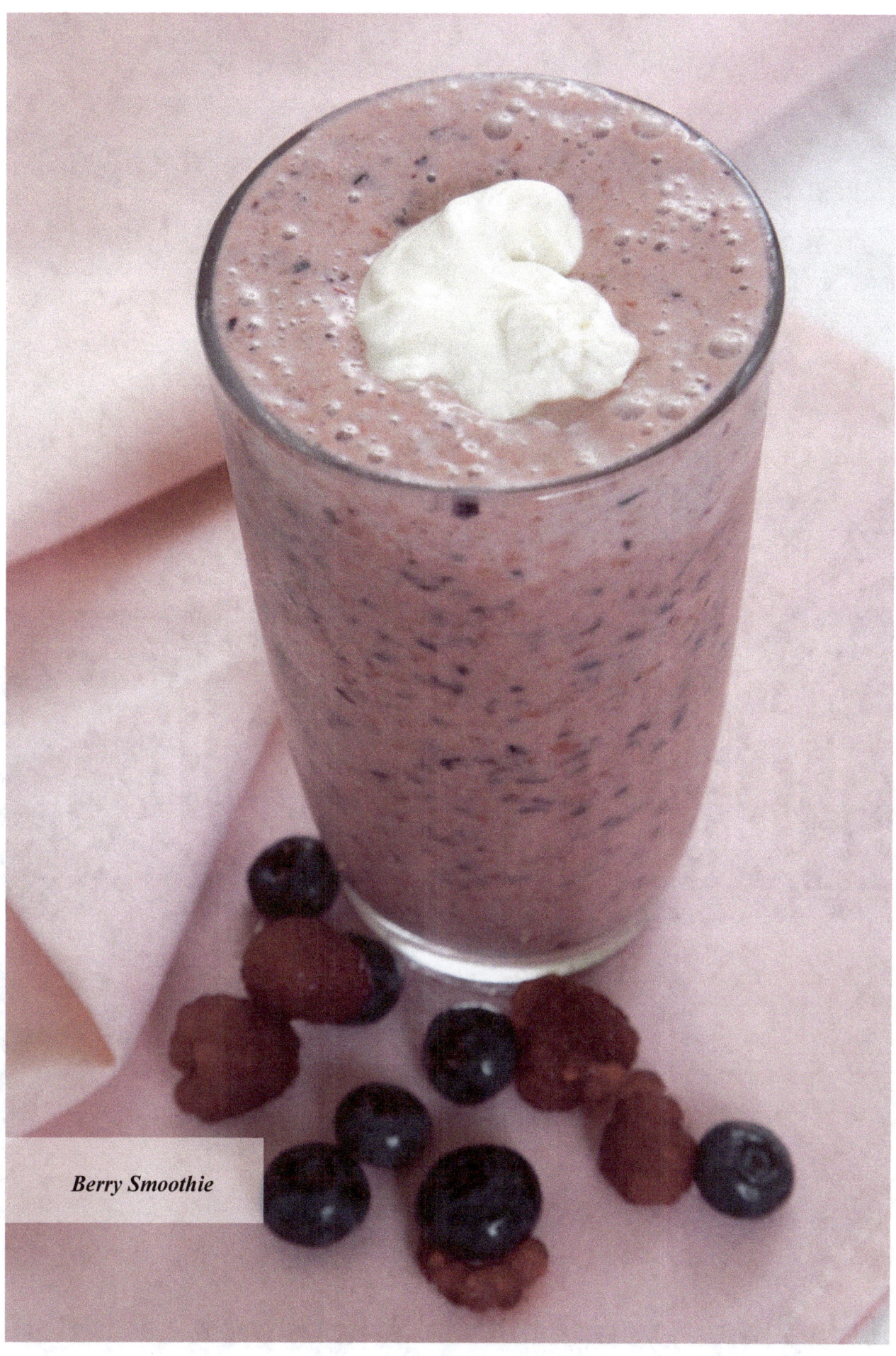

Berry Smoothie

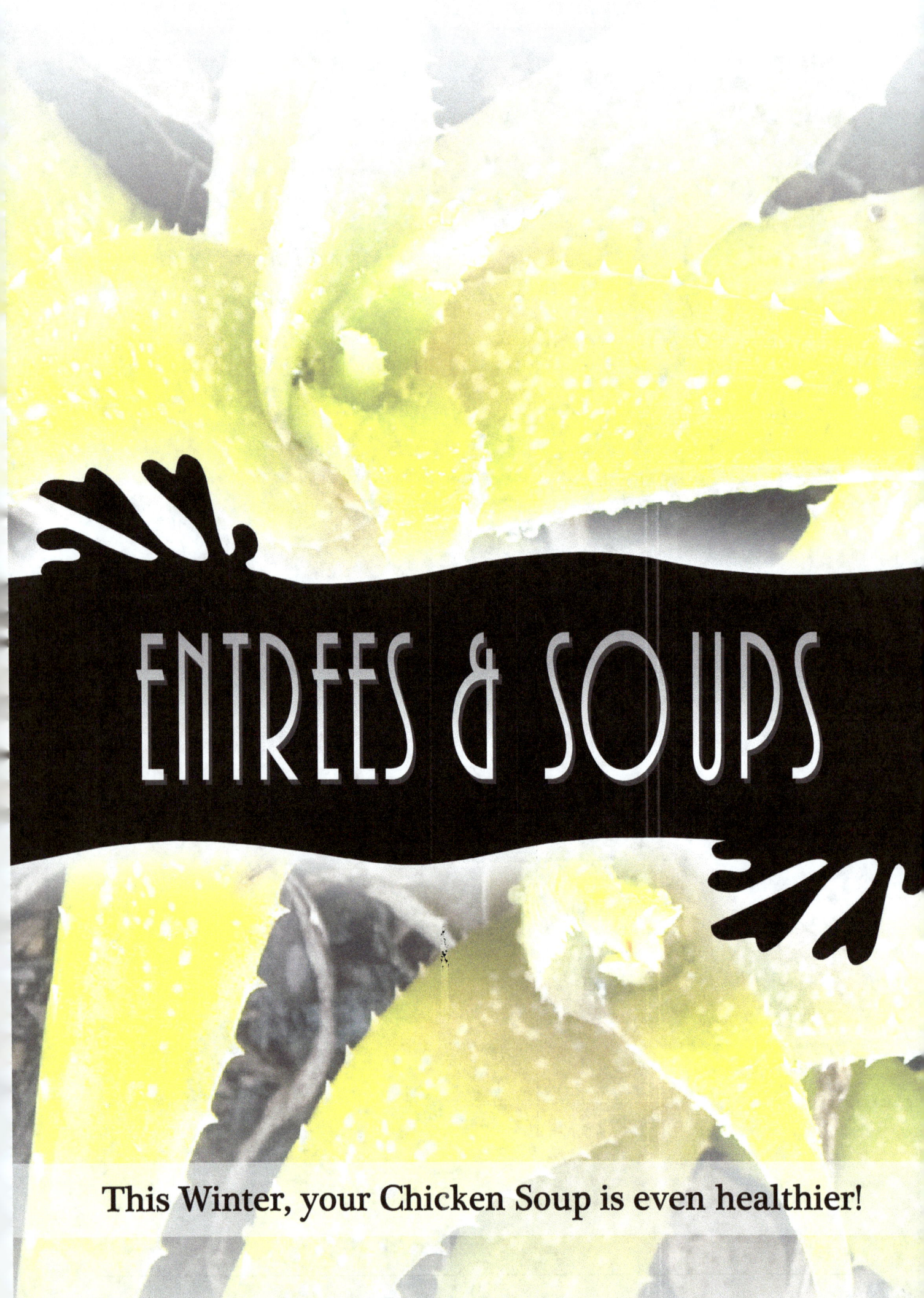

ENTREES & SOUPS

This Winter, your Chicken Soup is even healthier!

AVOCADO AND MANGO SAUCE

Ingredients
1 avocado
1 mango
1 Aloe vera leaf

Method
Cut avocado in half and scoop out of shell, place on plate cut and slice mango and put into a blender jug add Aloe vera gel and blend add salt and pepper to taste and pour over avocado half. Serves two.

VEGGIES AND PEANUT DIP

Ingredients

⅔ cup / 170ml water	⅓ cup / 100g smooth peanut butter
1 red capsicum	2 stalks of celery
1 clove of garlic	8 radishes
2 tspns ginger	2 spring onions
2 tblspns soy sauce	6 large carrots
chilli powder to taste	1 tblspn lemon juice
salt and pepper to taste	1 Aloe vera leaf

Method
Fry garlic and ginger then add the water in a saucepan. Stir in peanut butter, spring onion, soy sauce, chilli powder, salt and pepper. Simmer for two minutes and let cool. Then add the lemon and Aloe vera juice once the dip is cool, and you are ready to serve it up. Peel the carrots. Cut all the vegetables into small stick lengths. This is a great way to get the kids to enjoy eating raw veggies as they really love the dip, but you may have to remind them not to eat the dip on its own.

TAHINI DIP

Ingredients

¼ cup of Tahini paste	1 tblspn of honey
2 cloves of roasted garlic	4 tblspns of water
salt and pepper	1 blended Aloe vera leaf

Method
If serving straight away, put all the ingredients together in a bowl and mix well. Otherwise, prepare and mix in the Aloe vera just before serving the chilled Tahini.

Avocado and Mango Sauce

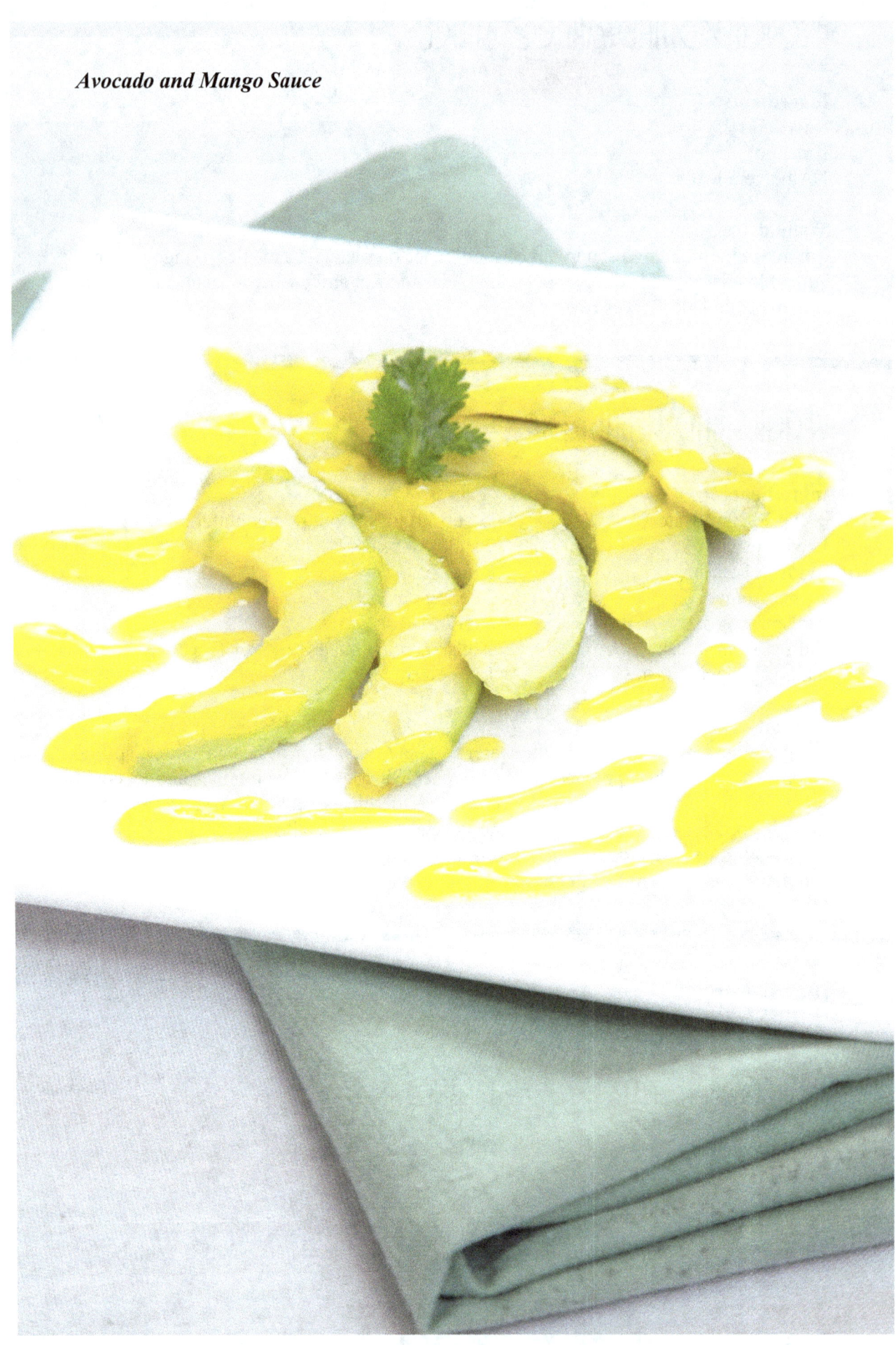

CHERRY TOMATOES WITH STUFFED PESTO

Ingredients

20 cherry tomatoes
1½ cups fresh basil
4 tblspns pumpkin seeds
2 cloves garlic
¼ cup water
3 tblspns olive oil
salt and pepper
1 Aloe vera leaf

Method

To make the pesto put all the ingredients into a blender scrape the Aloe gel into the blender too if serving immediately. Otherwise, mix blended Aloe into the pesto before serving. When cutting tops of cherry tomatoes you can put the pulp of the tomato into the pesto then spoon some pesto into each cherry tomato. All *Cookin' for Cures* dips can be served with pita bread and or raw vegetables.

EGGPLANT DIP

Ingredients

200g (7oz / 0.4lb) eggplant oven roasted
3 cloves of roasted garlic
1/2 lemon juiced
2 tspns Tahini paste
salt and pepper
1 tblspn olive oil
1 Aloe vera leaf

Method

After roasting the eggplant and garlic, skin eggplant and place in food processor for 1-2 minutes then add the roasted garlic, lemon juice, Tahini, oil salt, pepper and also Aloe leaf if using straight away. . Otherwise, mix in blended Aloe before serving. Blend ingredients for 1 to 2 minutes or until smooth. Aloe can be ready-made into a juice with the blender, and mixed in for serving - just make sure it is mixed through thoroughly.

TOASTED BREAD AND GARLIC MUSHROOMS

Ingredients

sour bread
2 cloves of garlic
fresh mushrooms
BBQ sauce
tasty and mozzarella cheese
1 Aloe vera leaf

Method

Fry mushrooms in a little oil with garlic and BBQ sauce add salt and pepper to taste. Add Aloe after finished cooking and place on bread sprinkle with cheese and lightly grill for a couple of minutes. Toast the sour bread and cover with mushrooms.

Cherry Tomato with stuffed Pesto

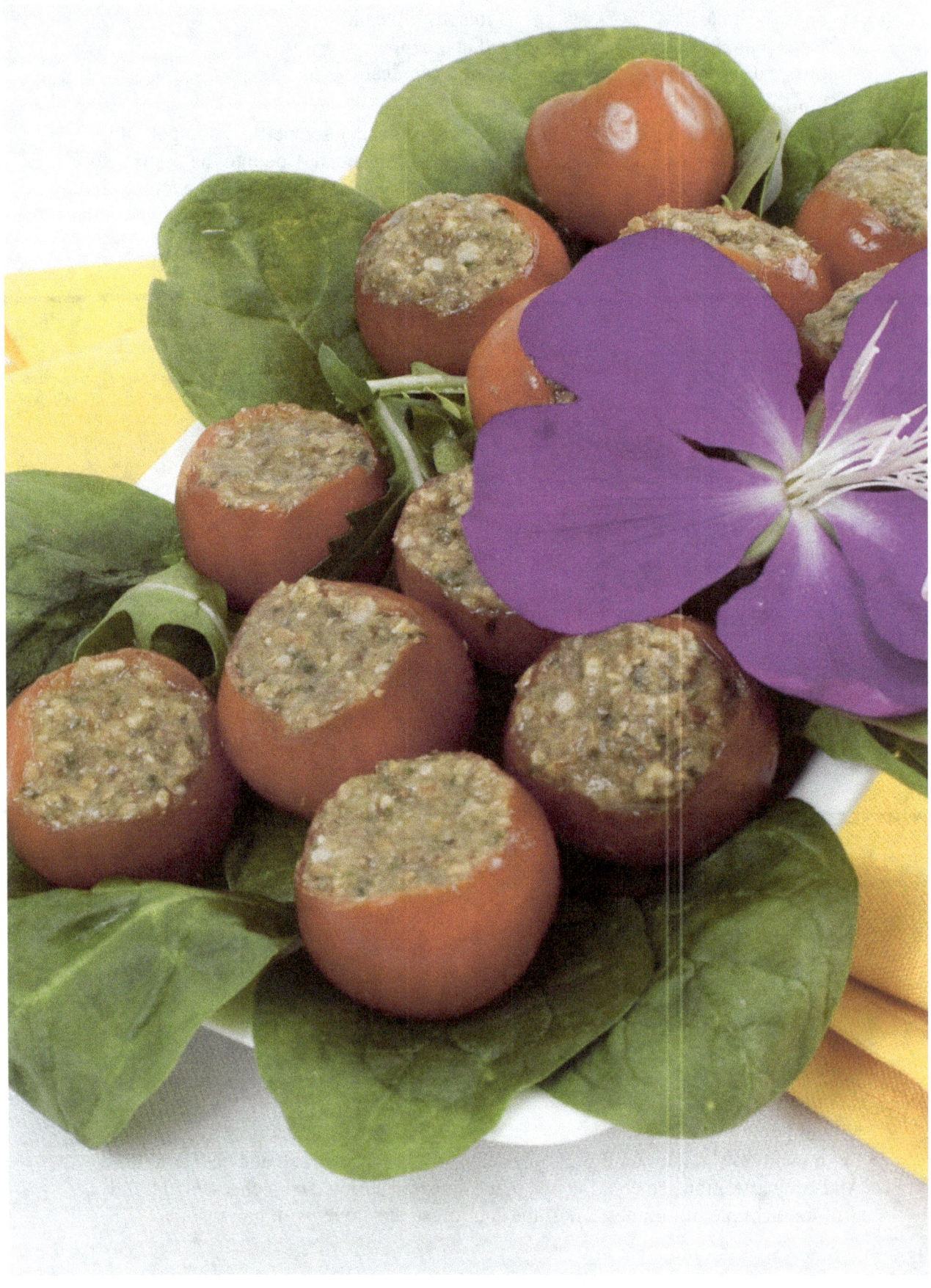

CHICKEN AND FIVE BEAN WRAP

Ingredients

500g (18oz) chicken pieces cubed
1 tin five beans
1 onion
2 chopped tomatoes
1 grated carrot
finely chopped lettuce
sour-cream
1 tspn cumin
1 tspn rosemary
grated tasty cheese to taste
salt and pepper to taste
flat wrap
1 Aloe vera leaf

Method

Fry onion in small quantity of oil. Add chicken and lightly brown then put in five beans and diced tomatoes. Cook for a few minutes until chicken is ready. Add cumin, rosemary, salt and pepper. Take off heat and add blended Aloe vera. Put all ingredients on table and each person can apply their own desired quantity.

PUMPKIN AND APPLE SOUP

Ingredients

Olive oil
1 onion
3 cloves of garlic
1 tblspn ginger
750g (26oz) butternut pumpkin
250g (9oz) green apples
2 tspns of thyme leaves
1½ tspns chilli powder
¼ cup of sour cream
3 cups of chicken stock
salt and pepper to taste
2 Aloe vera leaves

Method

Put diced onion, crushed garlic, and ginger into a saucepan and cook for 2 minutes. Add thinly sliced pumpkin and cook until tender. Add apples, thyme leaves, salt and pepper to taste stir gently. Add the stock and 1½ cups of water bring to boil and turn down to simmer for 30 minutes or until pumpkin is soft. Then place in processor with Aloe vera gel from two leaves and puree. Serve with a sprinkle of fresh thyme and chilli powder for those who like a little heat.

CREAMY CHICKEN SOUP

Ingredients

1 chicken carcass
1 onion
2 carrots
2 Aloe vera leaves
2 celery stalks
2 cups frozen corn
2 tblspns flour
1 tspn chilli (optional)
1 tspn mixed herbs
salt and pepper

Method

Place chicken carcass in saucepan and cover with water, heat for 30 minutes on a low setting. Then remove carcass from saucepan and scrape all the chicken off the body. Place onion in fry pan and cook until yellow. Place onion, chicken meat, carrots and celery back into the saucepan liquid. And simmer for 20-30 minutes. Then add herbs, salt, pepper and flour to thicken if you wish and blend all the soup into a smooth liquid and add blended Aloe vera juice to soup just before serving make sure it is well stirred in first.

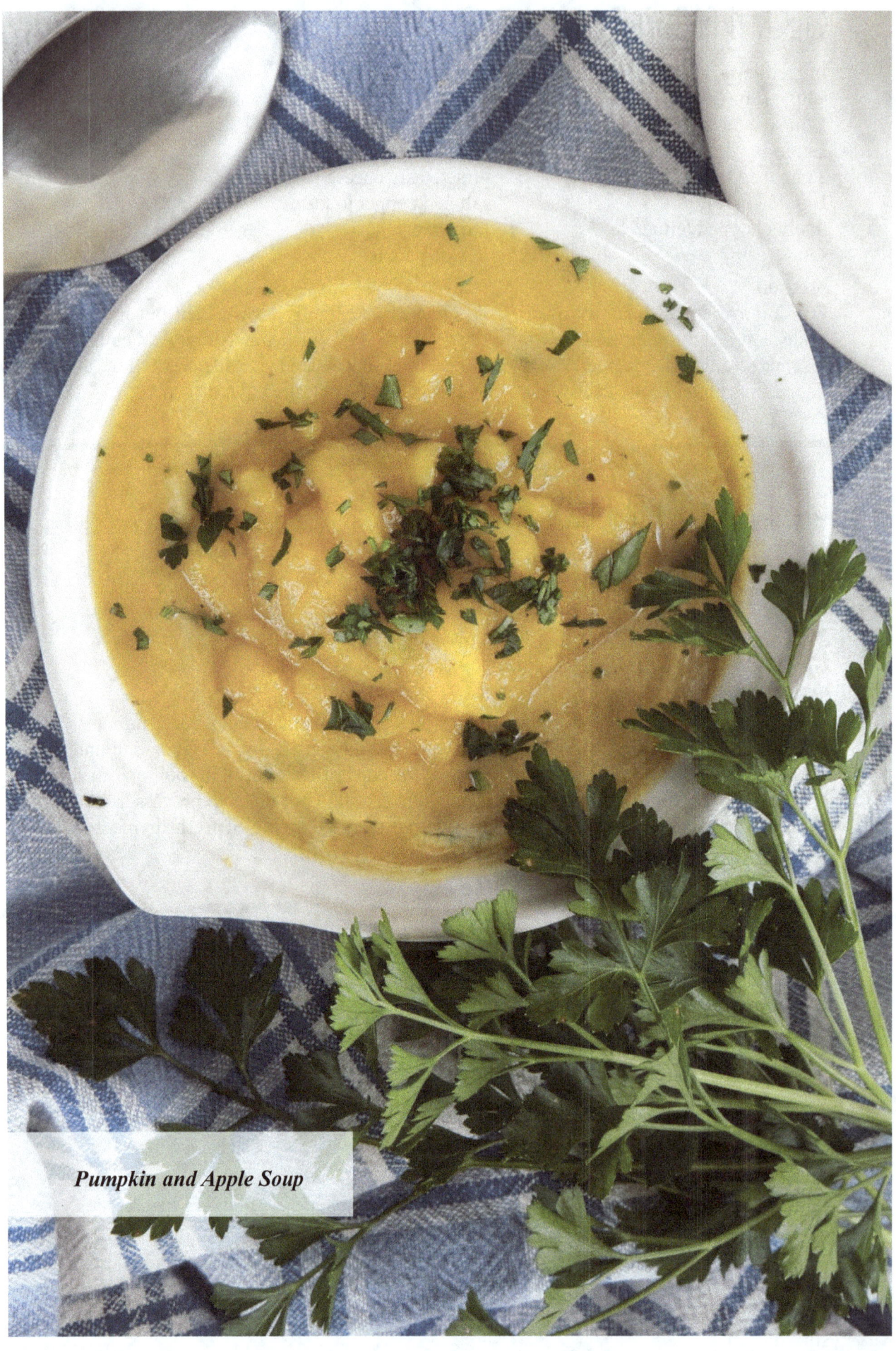
Pumpkin and Apple Soup

CREAM OF BROCCOLI SOUP

Ingredients
500g (18oz) broccoli
4 cups of vegetable Stock
pinch of basil
300g (10½oz) light cream cheese
salt and pepper to taste
1 Aloe vera leaf blended

Method
Cook broccoli in stock for ten minutes take off the heat and add salt, pepper, basil, cheese and blended Aloe vera leaf and serve immediately with bread.

CREAMY VEGETABLE SOUP

Ingredients

1 onion
1 carrot diced
1 cup of diced celery
4 cups of vegetable stock
½ cup of evaporated milk
1 Aloe vera leaf blended

Olive oil
1 cup of diced potato
4 cup of raw asparagus
2 tblspns of coriander
salt and pepper to taste

Method
In a large saucepan, sauté onion until soft. Add carrot, potato and celery. Cook on a low heat for around 10 minutes. Add rice and cover vegetable stock and cook for another 10 minutes. Add asparagus and simmer until tender. Turn off heat, add the milk, coriander and blended Aloe vera gel then serve with bread.

MINESTRONE SOUP

Ingredients

1L (1000ml / 34fl oz) stock
1 onion
½ a bacon rasher
salt, pepper and mixed herbs
1 carrot
1 turnip
1 stalk celery
2 handfuls cauliflower

2 cups of frozen corn
2 cups of peas
2 handfuls of beans chopped
¾ cup rice
1 tin tomatoes
2 Aloe vera leaves blended
2 tblspns of corn flour
1 pinch of chilli powder (optional)

Method
Fry onion in saucepan with diced bacon, add stock, salt, pepper, herbs and all veggies except beans, peas and corn. Cook for 1 hour and then add rice and beans, peas and corn. Cook for a further 10 minutes. Add salt, pepper and mixed herbs and adjust for your preferred flavour and thickness. Once you have taken off the heat, add in blended Aloe vera gel and stir in well.

Cream of Broccoli Soup

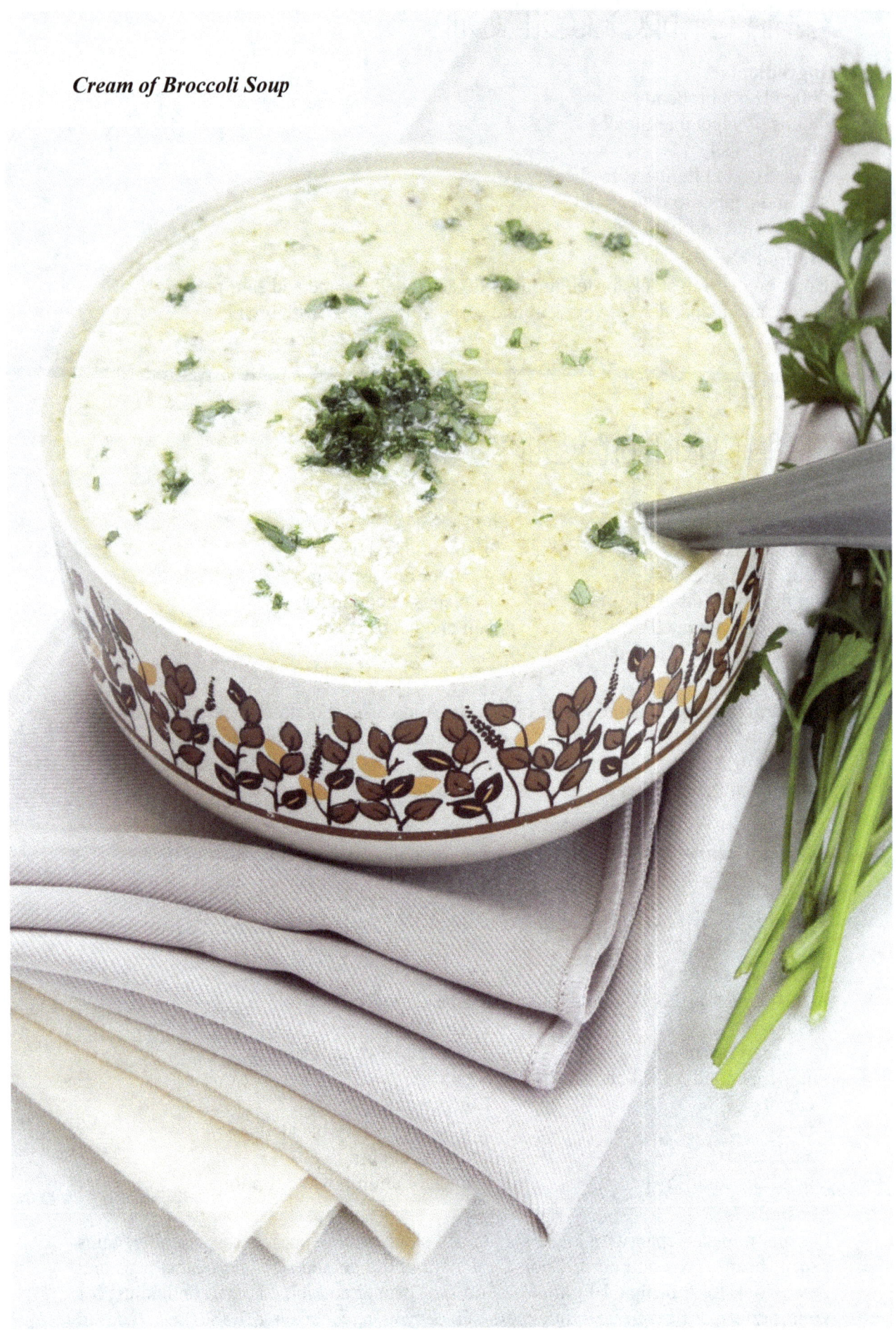

CHEESY CORN CHOWDER

Ingredients

2 rashers bacon (diced)
1 onion
1 stalk celery
2 cups (3 or 4 florets) cauliflower
salt and pepper
1 cup chicken stock liquid
2 tblspn flour
2 cups milk
2 cups frozen corn
1 tblspn red peppers
1 cup grated cheese
1 tblspn chopped parsley
2 Aloe vera leaves

Method

Lightly fry bacon, onion and celery in saucepan. Add cauliflower cook for two minutes. Add salt, pepper and chicken stock. Simmer until veggies are lightly cooked 7-10 minutes. Blend flour to ½ cup of milk stir until boiling and cook for 3 minutes. Add corn, red peppers cheese and parsley. Add more salt and pepper if needed. Take off heat and add Aloe vera Gel after blending, to the soup, mix well and serve with croutons or garnish.

THAI PRAWN SOUP

Ingredients

6 cups of fish stock
3 stalks of lemon grass tender white part crushed and cut into 2mm (0.1") slices
2 lime leaves
150g (5½oz) small mushrooms
4-6 fresh chillies seeded sliced
4 spring onions
2 tspns red curry paste
1 cup coriander leaves
2 tblspns fish sauce
8 large green prawns
½ cup lime juice
1 tblspn sugar
1 Aloe vera leaf

Method

Bring stock to boil in a large saucepan add lemon grass, lime leaves, mushrooms, fish sauce and chillies boil for 2 minutes. Then add the prawns, spring onions lime juice, sugar to the saucepan and cook for 2 minutes until the prawns are pink. Turn off the heat and add the coriander and the blended Aloe vera and serve straight away.

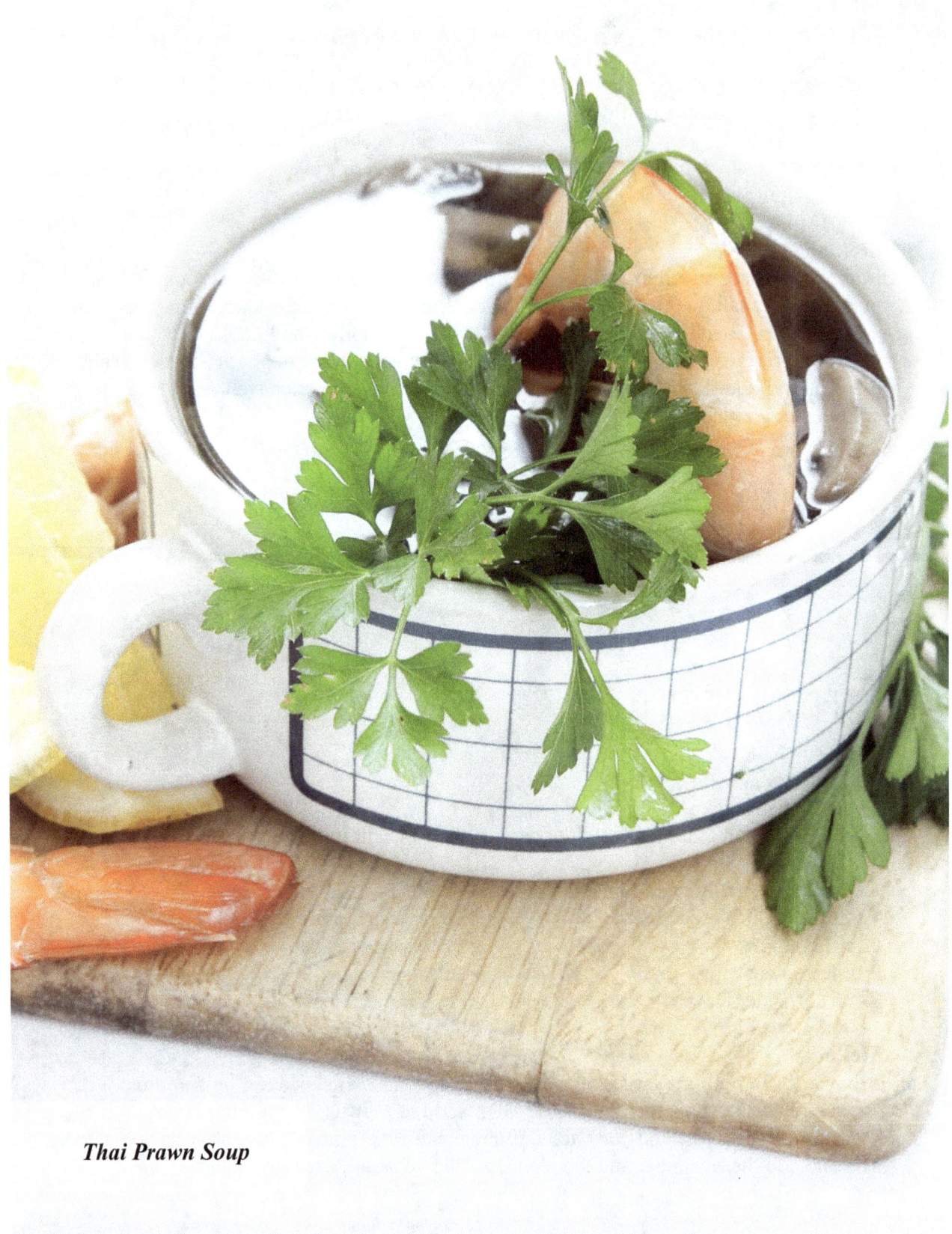

Thai Prawn Soup

MIXED SEAFOOD SOUP

Ingredients
4 good size spring onions
55g (2oz) noodles
2 tblspns of oil
2½cm (1") fresh ginger
75g (2½oz) small mushrooms
1¼L (1200ml / 40½fl oz) chicken stock
2 tblspns light soy sauce
125g (4½oz) mixed seafood - prawns, squid, scallops
75g (2½oz) bean sprouts
Fresh coriander leaves
1 Aloe vera leaf

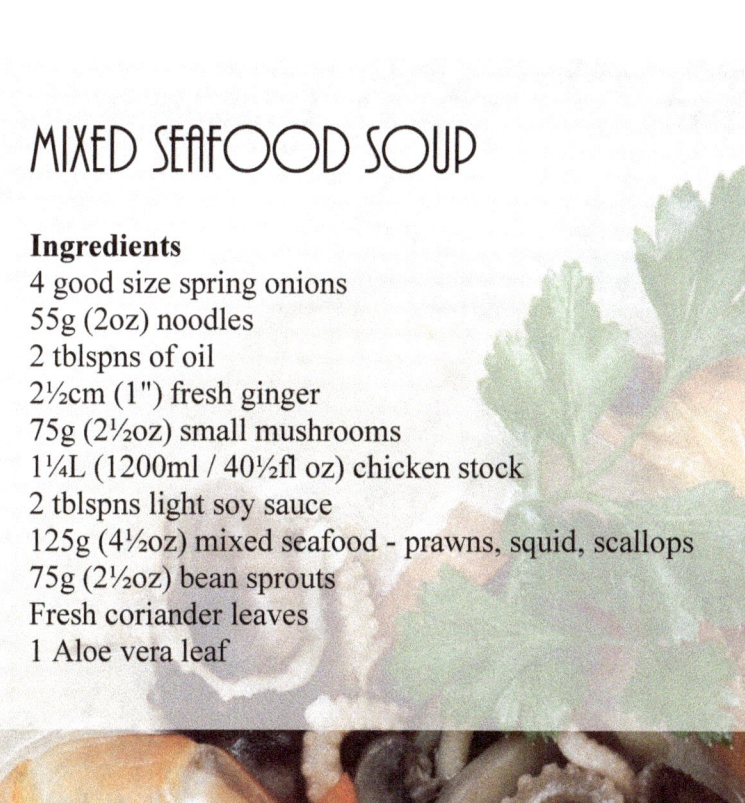

Method
Place noodles in a bowl and pour boiling water leave for 4 minutes. Put oil in fry pan and heat mushrooms and ginger once softened add stock soy sauce spring onions and bean sprouts and bring to boil. Add the mixed seafood and cook unit all is heated through. Drain the noodles and add bring back to boil and turn off the heat and add the blended Aloe vera gel. Then serve immediately.

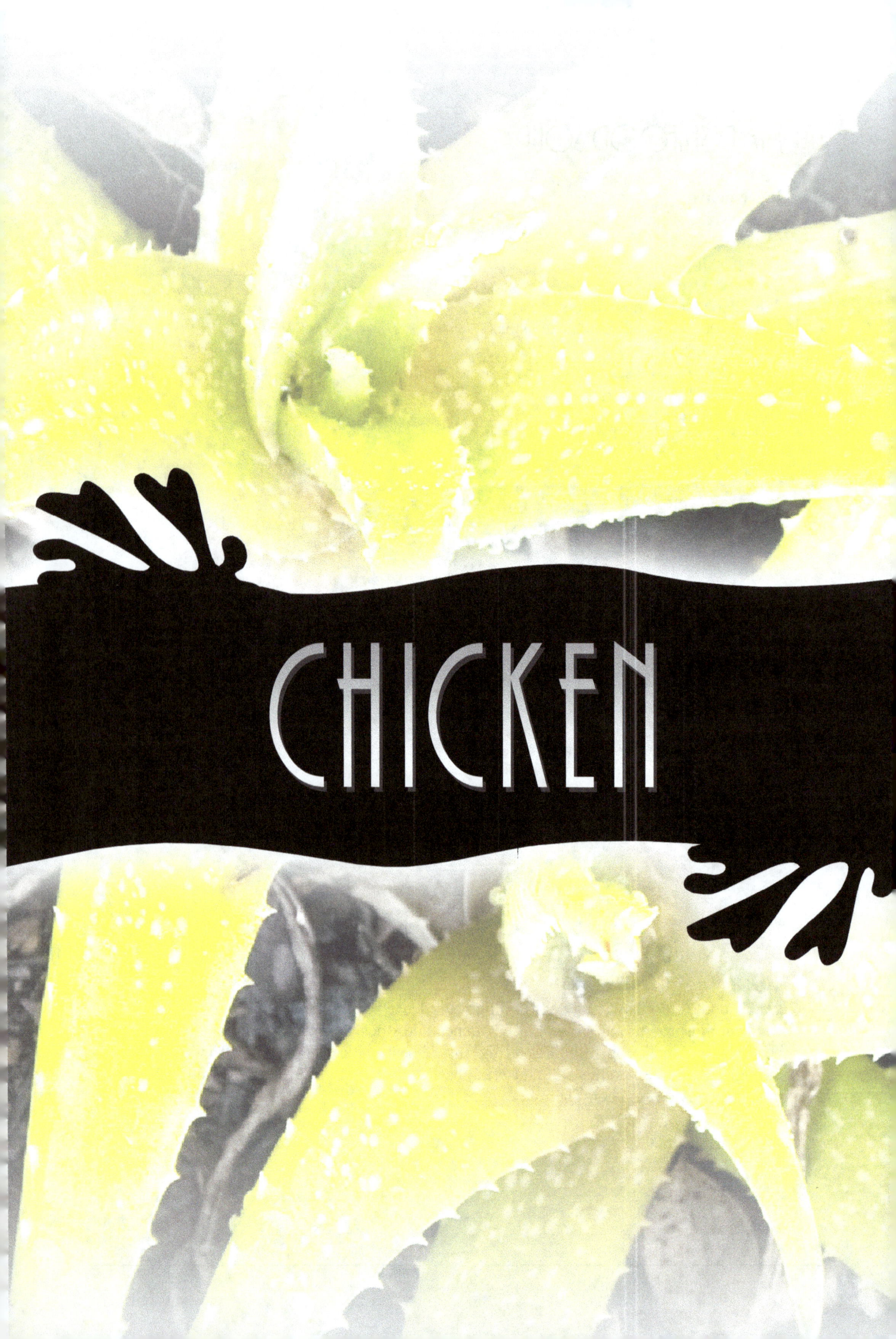

CHICKEN

GRILLED CHICKEN IN CHILLI AND MANGO SAUCE

Ingredients

1 medium skinless chicken breast
1 tbsp sweet chilli sauce
chopped parsley
¼ cup of chicken stock
1 cup mango puree
1 fresh mango (sliced and diced)
2 tblspns flour
1 Aloe vera leaf

Method

Trim fat from the chicken breast and slice length ways place in heated oiled pan. And brown both sides, do not cook all the way through. Remove from pan. Add mango puree and sweet chilli sauce to pan, add flour and chicken stock. Then reduce to simmer and place chicken in sauce, and heat through.

Place chicken on a plate and then add Aloe juice and parsley to the sauce after it has been taken off the heat. Then drizzle the sauce over the chicken and sprinkle a little more parsley over the chicken. Then add salad and fresh mango sliced and diced to the plate.

TANDOORI CHICKEN RIBS

Ingredients

1 kilo chicken ribs
1 tblspn cumin
1 tspn coriander
1 tspn fresh ginger
1 Aloe vera leaf
1 tblspn coriander
1 tspn chilli powder
3 cloves of garlic
½ cup of mango juice

Method

Blend all spices and juices together place in a plastic bag with the chicken ribs and make sure all the ribs are covered well with the tandoori marinade leave for ½ an hour and then cook on grill.

Place on boiled rice.

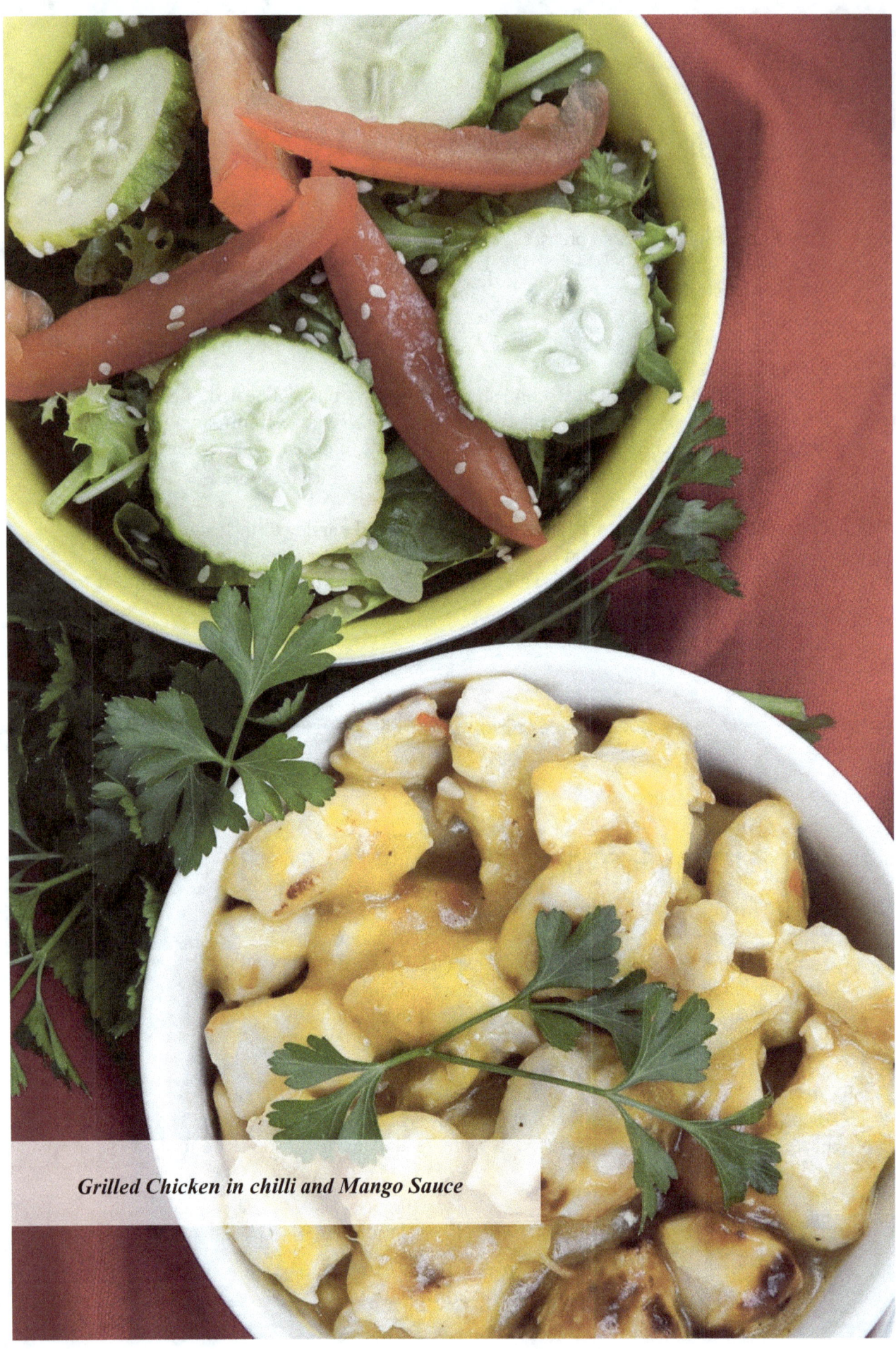

Grilled Chicken in chilli and Mango Sauce

GRILLED CHICKEN IN YOGHURT MARINADE

Ingredients

150g (5¼oz) / 4 chicken breast halves (skinless, boneless)
1 clove garlic
½ cup of low fat yoghurt
1 tblspn tomato paste
2 tspn ground cumin
1 tspn turmeric
1 tspn ginger
1 tspn chilli powder (optional)
salt and pepper
1 fresh coriander
1 Aloe vera leaf

Method

Combine crushed garlic, yoghurt, tomato paste, cumin, ground coriander, turmeric, chilli powder, ginger, fresh coriander, salt and pepper to taste, 1 blended Aloe vera Gel .Place chicken on a shallow dish and smother ingredients over the chicken and marinate for at least 1 hour. You can grill the chicken or pre heat the oven at 220°C (425°F). Place chicken in the oven rotate after fifteen minutes and remove after 30 minutes or when cooked through.

SATAY CHICKEN

Ingredients

1 tspn ginger
2 cloves garlic
2 large handfuls fresh coriander
½ lime zest
freshly chopped chilli
250g (9oz) toasted peanuts
2 Aloe vera leaves
1 tblspn fish oil
1 tblspn peanut oil
3 tblspns brown sugar
½ cup coconut cream
500g (18oz) chicken
1 tblspn soy sauce

Method

Crush ginger and garlic and place in puree blender, chop coriander, grate lime and chop chilli. Put in peanuts soy sauce and oils, sugar and cream and puree it all together. Place into a bowl with chicken pieces cut into cubes. Leave for at least an hour in the fridge to marinate. Just before cooking put blended Aloe vera gel into marinate and mix well then skewer all the meat. While cooking boil up some rice or make a nice citrus salad to go with it

Grilled Chicken in Yoghurt Marinade

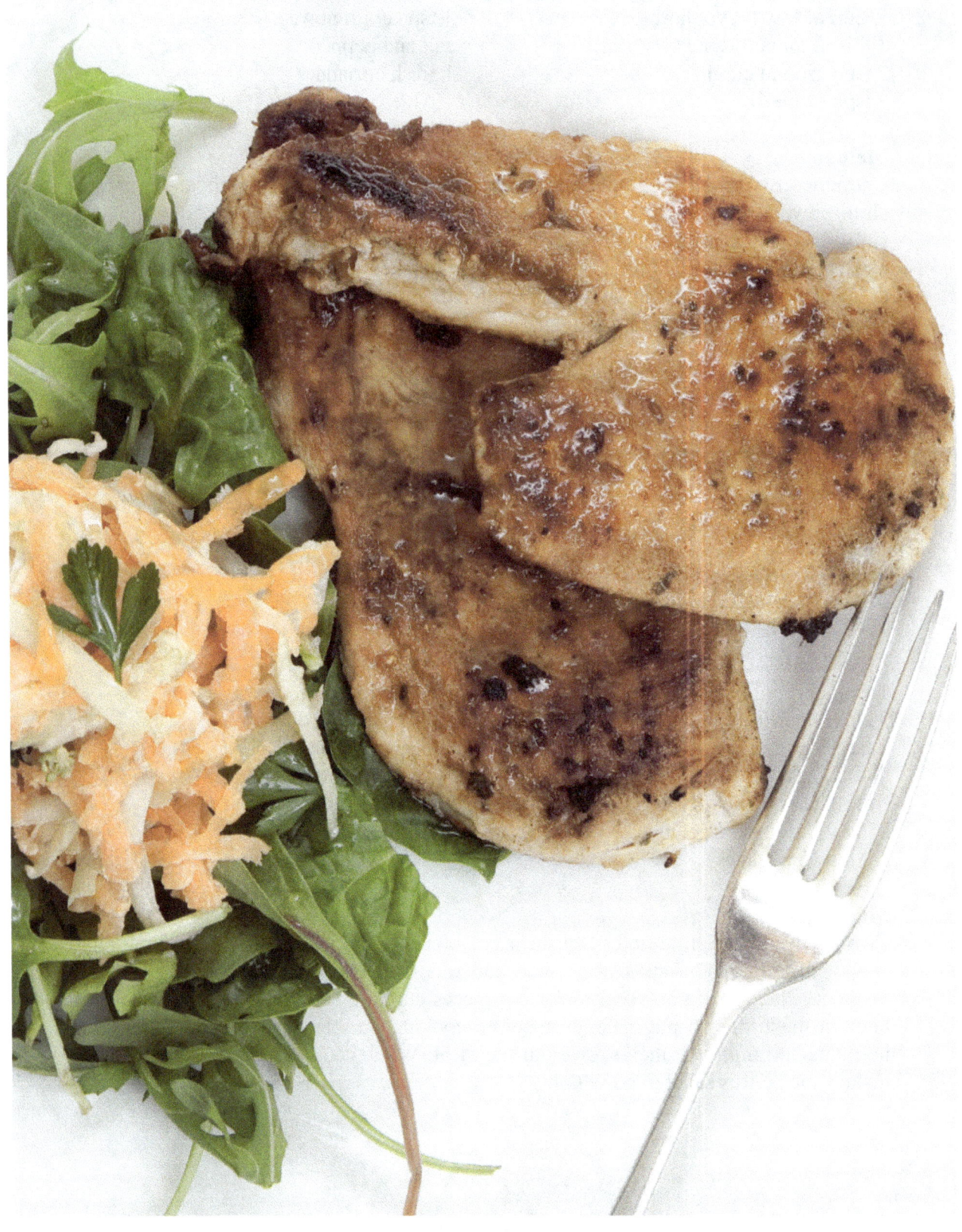

STIR FRY CHICKEN AND CASHEWS

Ingredients
375g (13oz) skinless, boneless chicken thighs cut small cubes
3 cups of broccoli
3 tspns of BBQ sauce
3 tspns of dry sherry (optional)
2 tspns cooking oil
3 tspns grated ginger
3 cloves of crushed garlic
1 red capsicum (pepper) diced
1 tblspn mixed herbs
2 tblspns chilli sauce
2 carrots thinly sliced
2 tblspns corn flour
2 spring onions sliced
¼ cup cashews
½ cup chicken stock
2 Aloe vera leaves

Method
Cook broccoli in a steamer for 3 minutes or until crisp-tender, put aside. Mix BBQ sauce and sherry in a bowl. Add the chicken and toss. Heat oil in a large fry pan. Add chicken and stir fry for three minutes. Transfer to a plate. Add ginger and garlic and onion stir fry for 30 seconds. Add the Broccoli, carrots and capsicum and stir fry for two minutes. Add stock and chilli sauce and bring to boil, Mix corn flour with a tblspn of cold water to make a paste, then add to pan and stir until slightly thickened. Return the chicken for one minute. Stir in cashews herbs and Aloe once heat is off.

CHICKEN AND BACON STIR FRY

Ingredients
500g (18oz) sliced chicken
1 onion
1 broccoli
1 tspn mixed herbs
3 tspns plain flour
¼ tspn chilli powder
1 Aloe vera leaf
6 rashers of bacon (diced)
3 medium size carrots
1 tspn rosemary
1 cup chicken stock
salt and pepper to taste
1 cup steamed rice

Method
Dice onions and place in fry pan with oil, add carrots and lightly cook. Add the chicken, bacon broccoli and the green beans mix until lightly cooked then add herbs, rosemary, flour, chicken stock, salt and pepper to taste and chilli powder. Serve with rice or mix rice into the fry pan stir in Aloe vera juice just before serving.

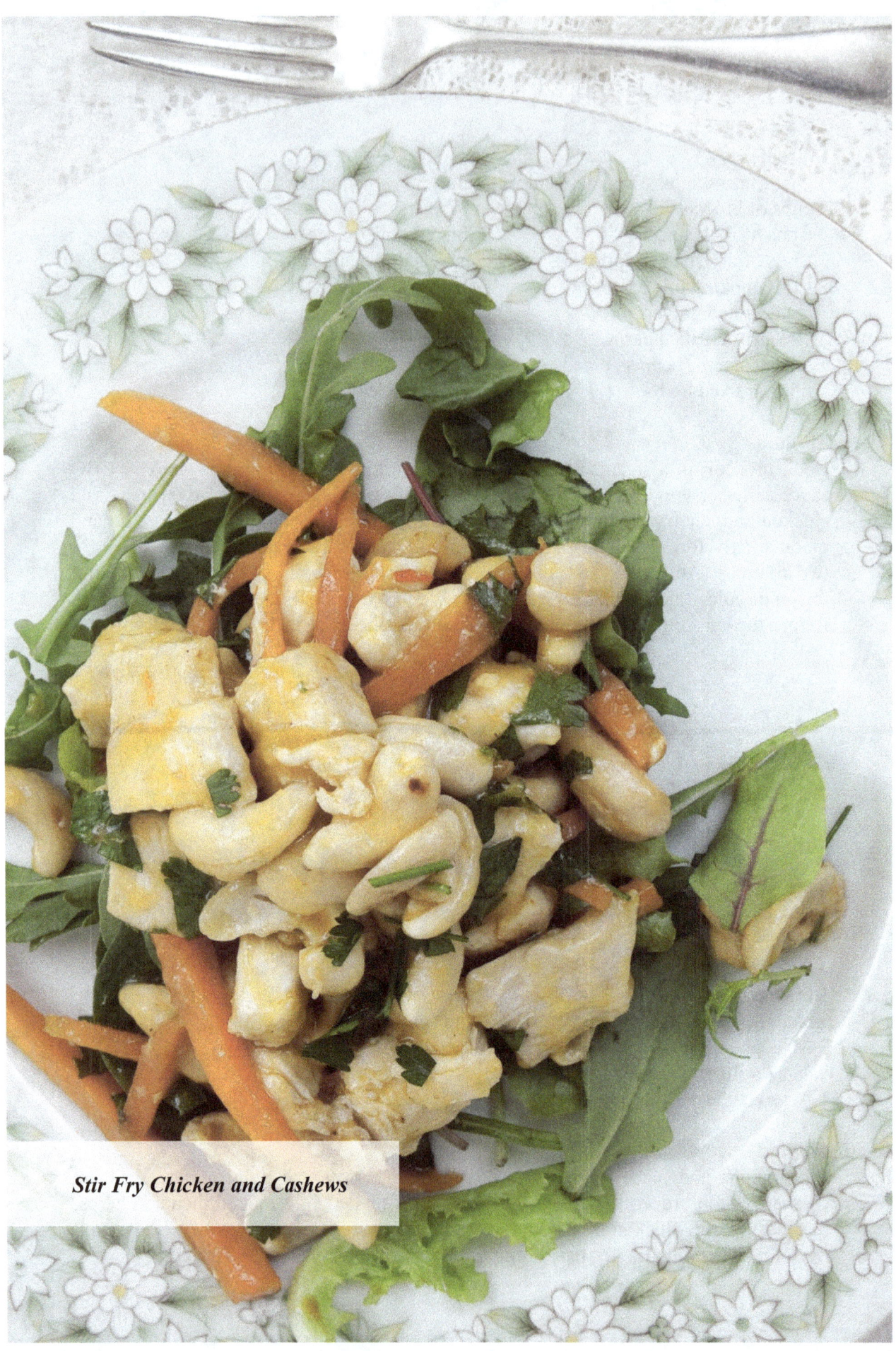
Stir Fry Chicken and Cashews

ROSEMARY AND ORANGE SAUCE OVER CHICKEN

Ingredients

600g (21oz) chicken breasts
4 tspns balsamic vinegar
1 clove garlic
spray of olive oil

2 oranges juiced
½ orange zest
2 tspns rosemary
1 Aloe vera leaf

Method

Trim breasts and place into shallow baking dish. Add juice zest rosemary garlic and vinegar and marinate for 30 minutes.

Grill chicken until cooked and remove from heat. Add marinate to pan juices and simmer for 5 minutes you can thicken slightly with flour and a little chicken stock if you wish and once taken off the heat add Aloe vera leaf and drizzle over meat and serve immediately.

BERRY AND MANDARIN GLAZED BREASTS

Ingredients

1 mandarin juice
100g (3½oz) strawberries
4 tblspns balsamic vinegar
1 clove of garlic
1 Aloe vera leaf

600g (21oz) chicken Breast
olive oil
2 mandarins
2 tblspns of sage leaves

Method

Blend berries juices and vinegar and push through a sieve and remove all the pith. Add garlic crushed 1 tblspn of sage and pour into a shallow dish. Add chicken and marinate for around 30 minutes.

Place leanly cut breasts in a lightly oiled oven proof dish and baste with marinate and place mandarin segment over the meat and lightly drizzle or spray with oil. Sprinkle with the remanding sage and bake for 15-20 minutes basting regularly when removed from oven put the blended Aloe vera into the last of the marinate stir well then drizzle generously over the fillet and serve.

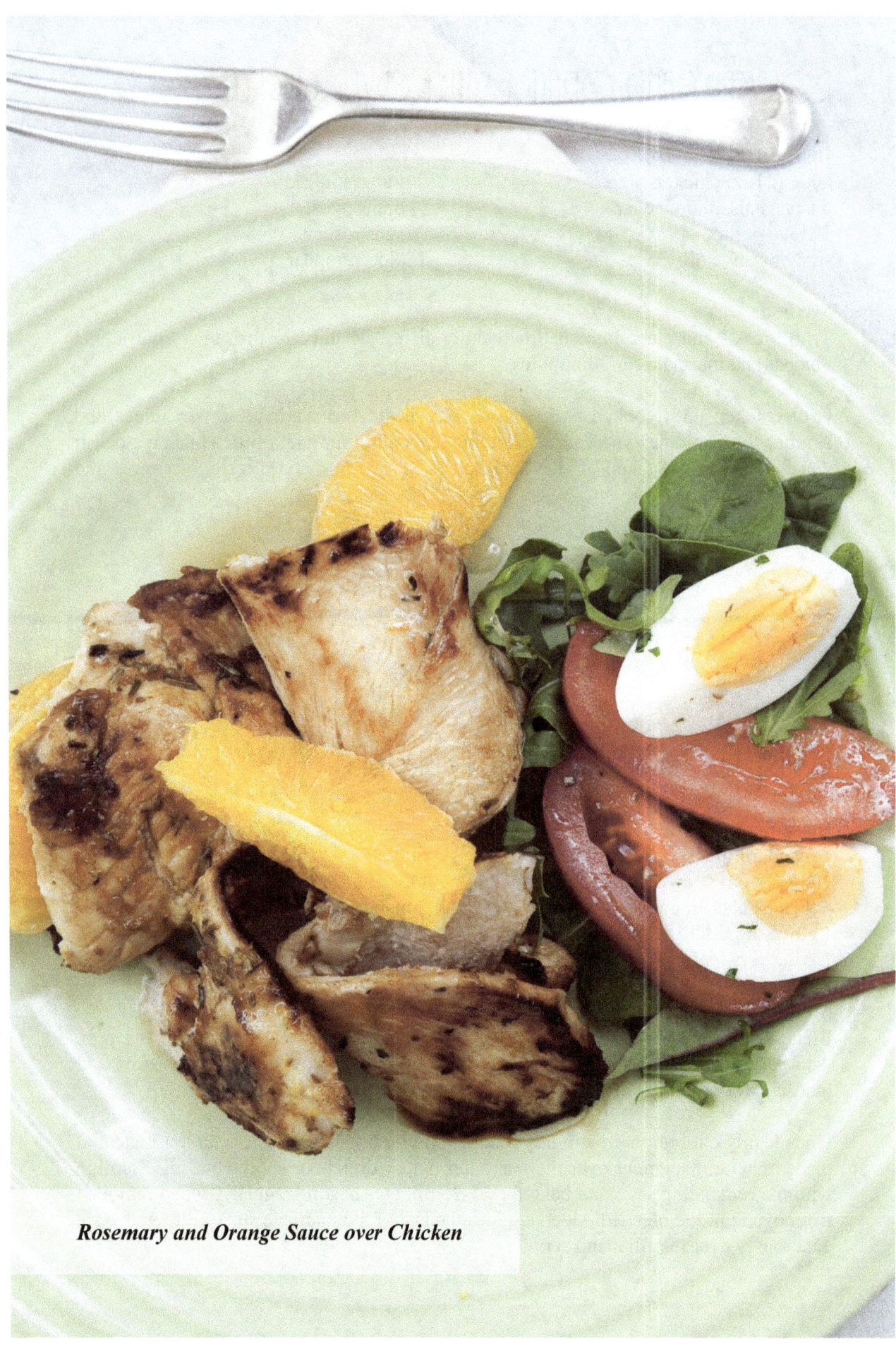

Rosemary and Orange Sauce over Chicken

CHICKEN PARMIGIANA

Ingredients

½ cup of parmesan
½ cup dry bread crumbs
2 eggs
2 tblspns tomato pasta sauce
4 skinless, boneless chicken breast
¼ cup of shredded mozzarella cheese
3 tspns olive oil
2 Aloe vera leaves

Method

Preheat oven to 220°C (425°F). Place the parmesan and the bread crumbs on some greaseproof paper on a tray place in the oven for a few minutes. Beat egg in a shallow bowl. Dip the chicken into the parmesan, then the egg white and 1 Aloe mixture, then into the breadcrumb. Heat oil in, a fry pan. Cook the chicken on both sides until lightly browned. (3 minutes). Place onto a baking tray spread blended tomato paste with Aloe vera and sprinkle with mozzarella and cook until cheese is a nice golden brown. Sever with veggies or a salad.

CHICKEN MEATLOAF

Ingredients

500g (17½oz) chicken mince
1 broccoli flower
1 carrot
1 parsnip
1 zucchini
3 cups corn
2 cups bread crumbs
3 chicken stock cubes
3 eggs
100g (3½oz) pine nuts
1 tblspn tarragon
1 tblspn sage
2 cups grated tasty cheese
3 tblspns plain flour
1 cup milk
1 Aloe vera leaf

Method

Grate all veggies then mix all the ingredients together well, flatten out in a baking dish and cover with foil and cook for 20 minutes at 250°C (425°F). Make a cheese sauce using cheese flour milk and Aloe vera, and put back in the oven for 10 minutes or until golden.

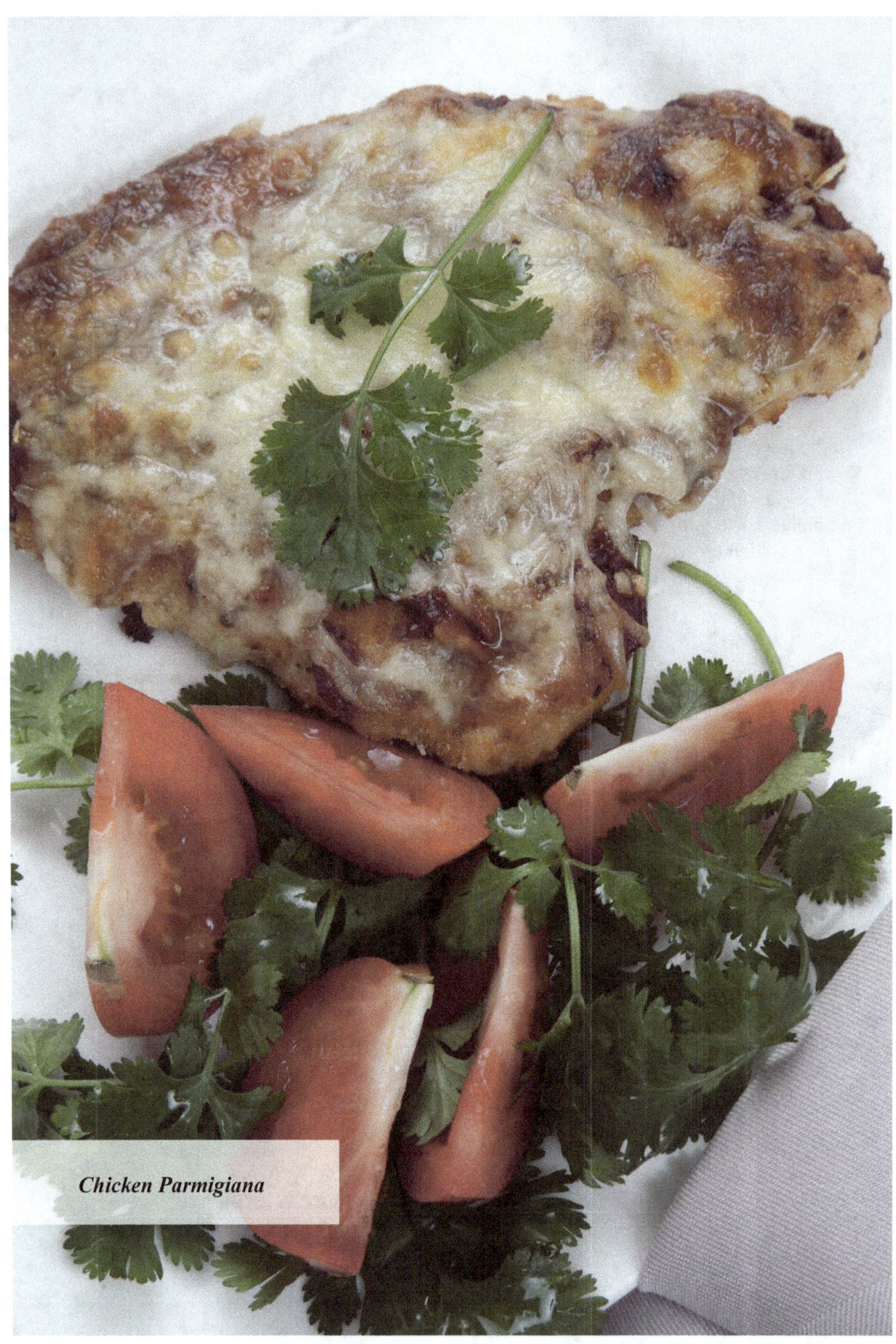

Chicken Parmigiana

CHINESE CHICKEN NOODLES

Ingredients

250g (9oz) spaghetti or linguine
1 tblspn soy sauce
1 tblspn white vinegar
2 carrots
1 red, green & yellow (pepper)
1 tblspn rosemary
1 tspn ginger
1 Aloe vera leaf

375g (13¼oz) cooked chicken breast
1 cup crushed almonds
1 dsrtspn sugar
3 tspns sesame oil
2 spring onion
2 cups chicken stock
salt and pepper

Method

Cook the pasta- spaghetti in boiling water until ready.
Meanwhile combine the soy, vinegar, sesame oil, sugar ginger, pinch of salt and pepper into large bowl. Toss shredded chicken; crushed Almonds, very thin slivered carrots and capsicum also add the blended Aloe vera gel and pasta or spaghetti. Toss all ingredients well and serve.

ROAST CHICKEN WITH VEGETABLES

Ingredients

1 chicken (trimmed of fat)
10 sprigs rosemary
1 tblspn sage leaves
6 large garlic cloves
4 carrots peeled

½ cup chicken stock
2 tblspns lemon juice
3 tblspns plain flour
2 Aloe vera leaves
4 potatoes

Method

Preheat oven 210°C (415°F). Stuff cavity with rosemary leaves save 2 tspns for later; also add sage and garlic to cavity. Place chicken breast in baking dish and bake for 30 minutes. Turn over and bake for a further 30 minutes. Put veggies in a separate dish and bake in the oven until golden brown. Transfer to plate.

Add the stock lemon, reserved rosemary leaves and ¼ cup of water and stir scraping the brown bits from the sides. Pour into gravy separator or place in freezer for 15 minutes and then scrape solid fat off the top. Pour gravy juices in with flour and ¼ cup water and place into a saucepan and cook over a medium heat, stirring until the gravy is thickened. Take off the heat add blended Aloe vera leaves and serve beside or over the chicken

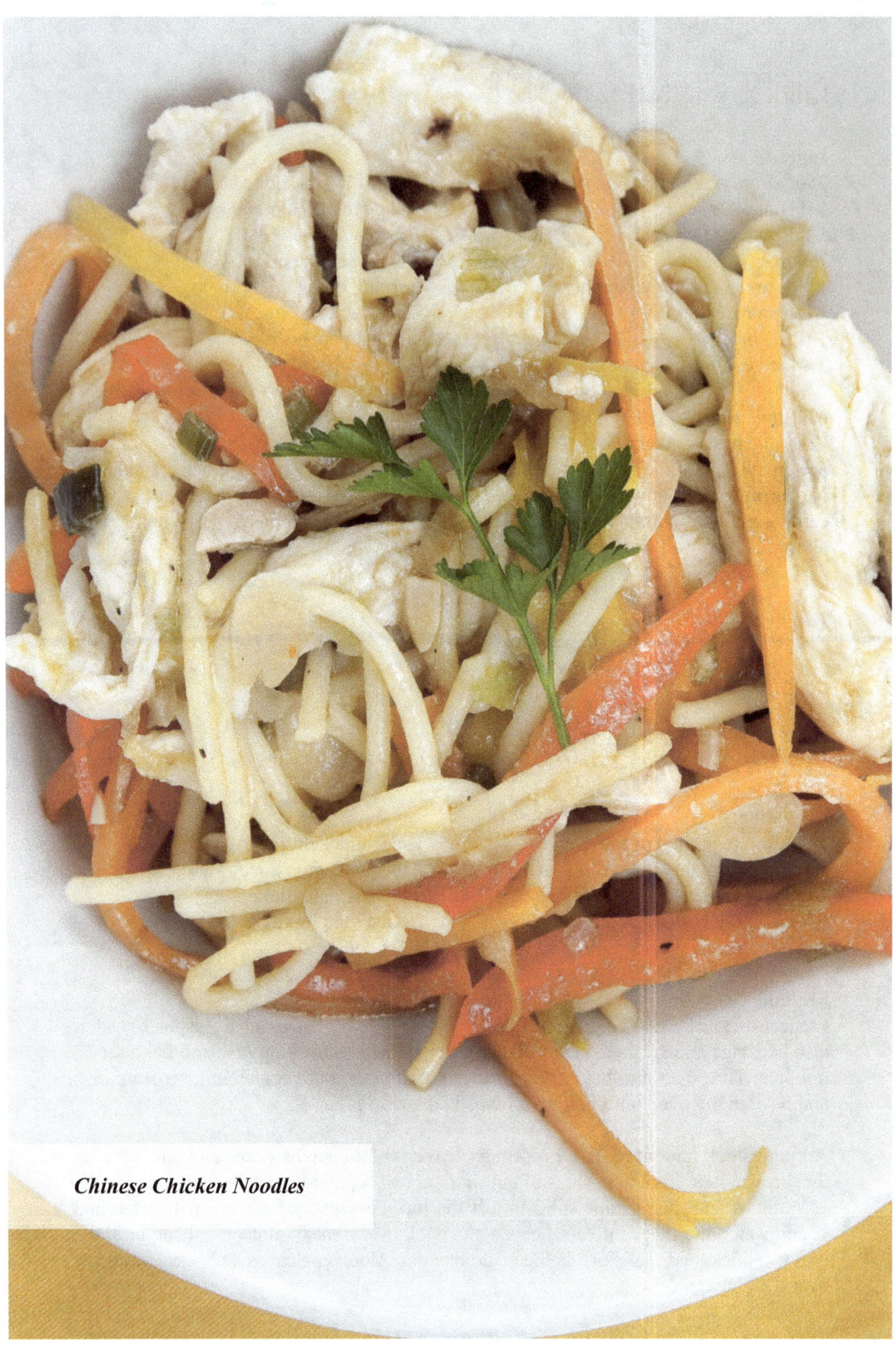

Chinese Chicken Noodles

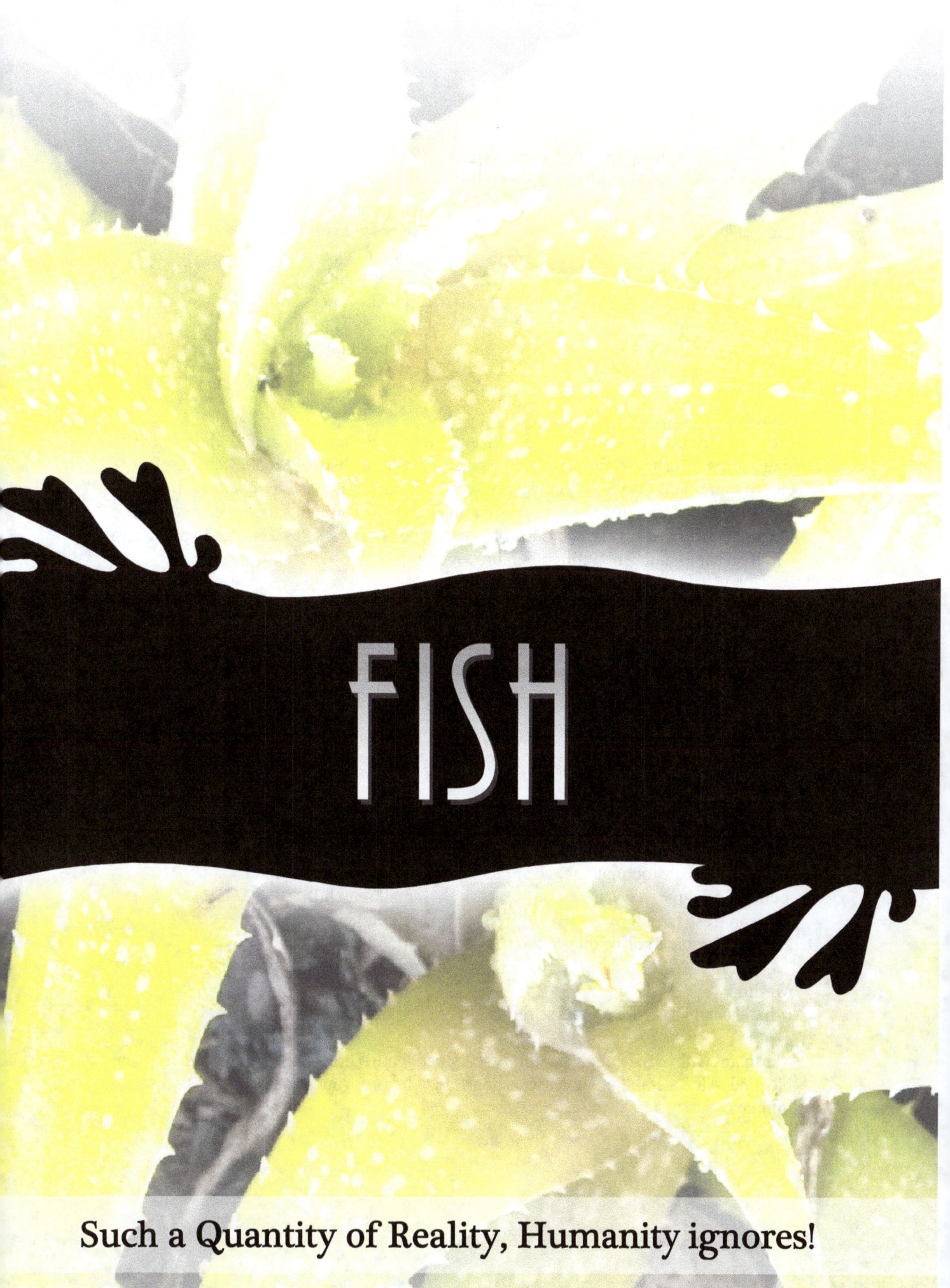

LOBSTER (CRAYFISH) MORNAY

Ingredients
1 crayfish (lobster, cooked)
1 preparation cheese sauce >
lemon slices
sprigs of parsley

Sauce Ingredients
1 cup of veggie stock
2 tblspns flour
salt and pepper
mixed herbs to taste
4 tblspns grated cheese
1 Aloe vera leaf

Method
Prepare crayfish (lobster) cut into half lengthways. Remove flesh and chop into bite size pieces. Wash crayfish shells and place in baking dish. To make Sauce, place 1 cup of either milk, water or veggie stock, in jug add cheese, salt, pepper and flour and stir well place in microwave and cook until it becomes a thick sauce. Leave to cool a little and then add Cray meat and blended Aloe, mix well together and spoon into Crayfish shells and grill until golden brown on top.

CHILLI BABY OCTOPUS

Ingredients
600g (21oz) baby octopus
4 cloves of garlic
1 tblspn fresh tarragon
20ml (1-2 capfuls) olive oil

large saucepan of water
1small red chilli
1 tblspn lemon
1 Aloe vera leaf

Method
If hoods and beaks are on please remove them and cut the octopi in half.

Marinate with crushed garlic finely chopped chilli oregano lemon olive oil and blended Aloe vera. For at least 1 hour. Just before you serve, char grill for two minutes.

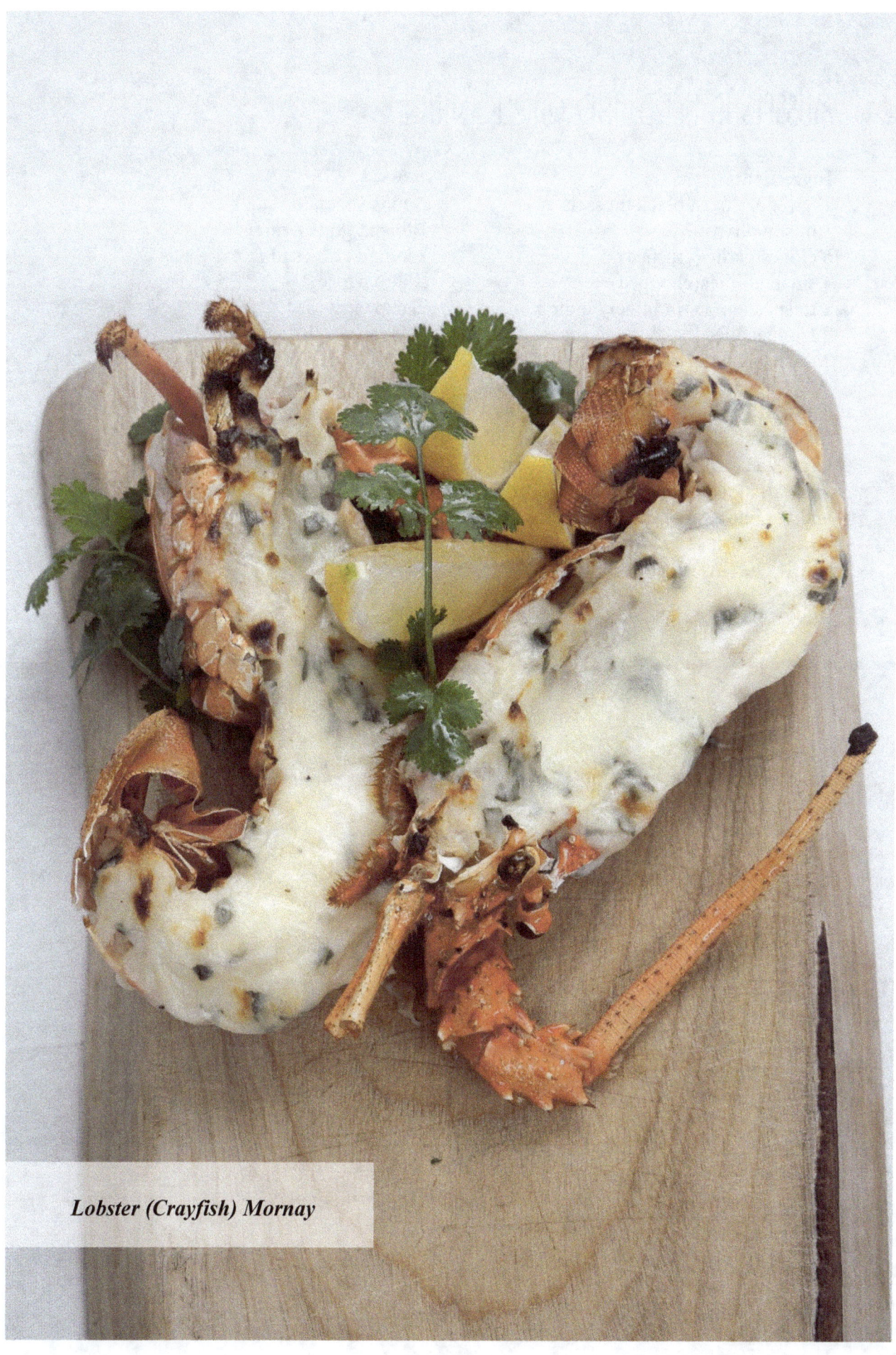

Lobster (Crayfish) Mornay

MUSSELS IN HERB AND GARLIC SAUCE

Ingredients

1kg (35oz) fresh black mussels
1 tblspn olive oil
6 cloves garlic (crushed)
4 small chillies (chopped)
2 tblspns lemon rind finely grated
2 lemons juiced
2 tblspns white wine vinegar
2 cups vegetable stock
1 tblspn grated ginger
2 lemon grass stalks
½ cup parsley
¼ cup basil
1 Aloe vera leaf

Method

De-beard and scrub mussels under cold water discard any that do not shut. Heat oil in large saucepan, add garlic, chilli, and lemon rind and stir for 1 minute. Add juice, vinegar, stock, ginger and lemon grass. Simmer for 10 more minutes. Take off heat and put into a large bowl add herbs and blended Aloe vera juice in and mix well.

BBQ SEAFOOD STICKS

Ingredients

4 prawns de-headed peeled and veined.
2 small thick fillets
4 scallops
1 lemon
2 tspns parsley
2 tspns paprika
salt and pepper
1 Aloe vera leaf

Method

Blend all marinated ingredients and add the fish, seafood and marinate for 30 minutes. Then skewer one of each on a skewer and grill on the barbeque. Goes well with a salad.

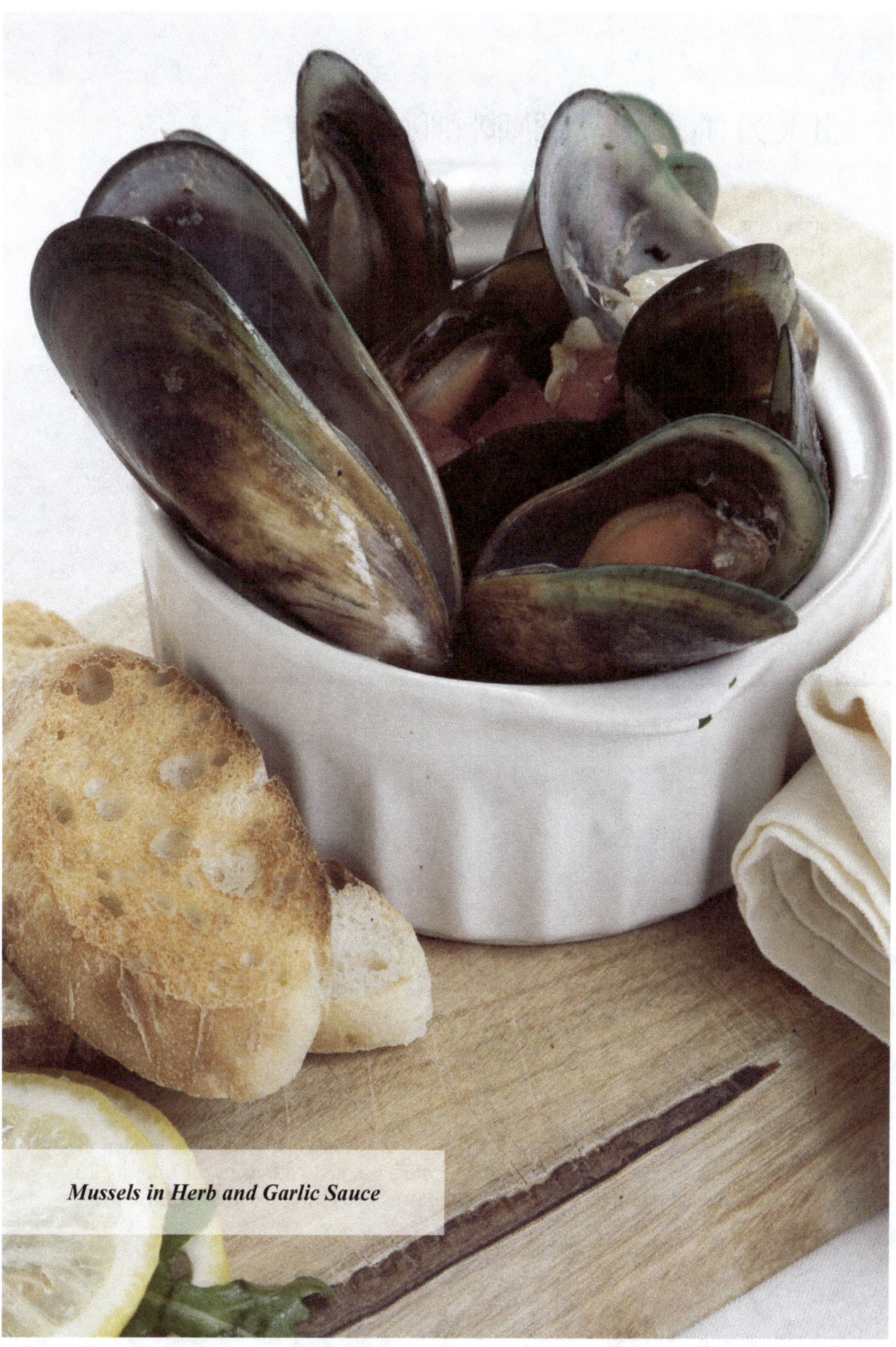
Mussels in Herb and Garlic Sauce

LEMON AND CHILLI CALAMARI BARBEQUED

Ingredients
600 grams (21oz) squid hoods
4 cloves garlic
2 small red chillies
2 lemons (juiced)
20ml (1-2 capfuls) olive oil
salt and pepper to taste
1 Aloe vera leaf

Method
Rinse the squid hoods and with a sharp knife cut into 1cm thick rings. Marinate calamari in bowl with garlic, chilli, lemon juice, oil pepper and blended Aloe vera leaf for 1 hour. Cook on BBQ for 2 minutes or until calamari is fully white.

BBQ PRAWNS

Ingredients
1kg (35oz) large fresh green prawns
10 cloves fresh garlic
salt and pepper
1 tblspn lemon thyme (herb)
1 tblspn olive oil
1 Aloe vera leaf

Method
Remove the prawn heads, de shell and cut prawns down the spine and remove the vein. Place garlic, salt pepper lemon thyme olive oil, and Aloe vera gel from its leaf into a blender and mix well. Place paste on prawns in a bowl mix well and sit for ½ an hour. BBQ for 2 minutes.

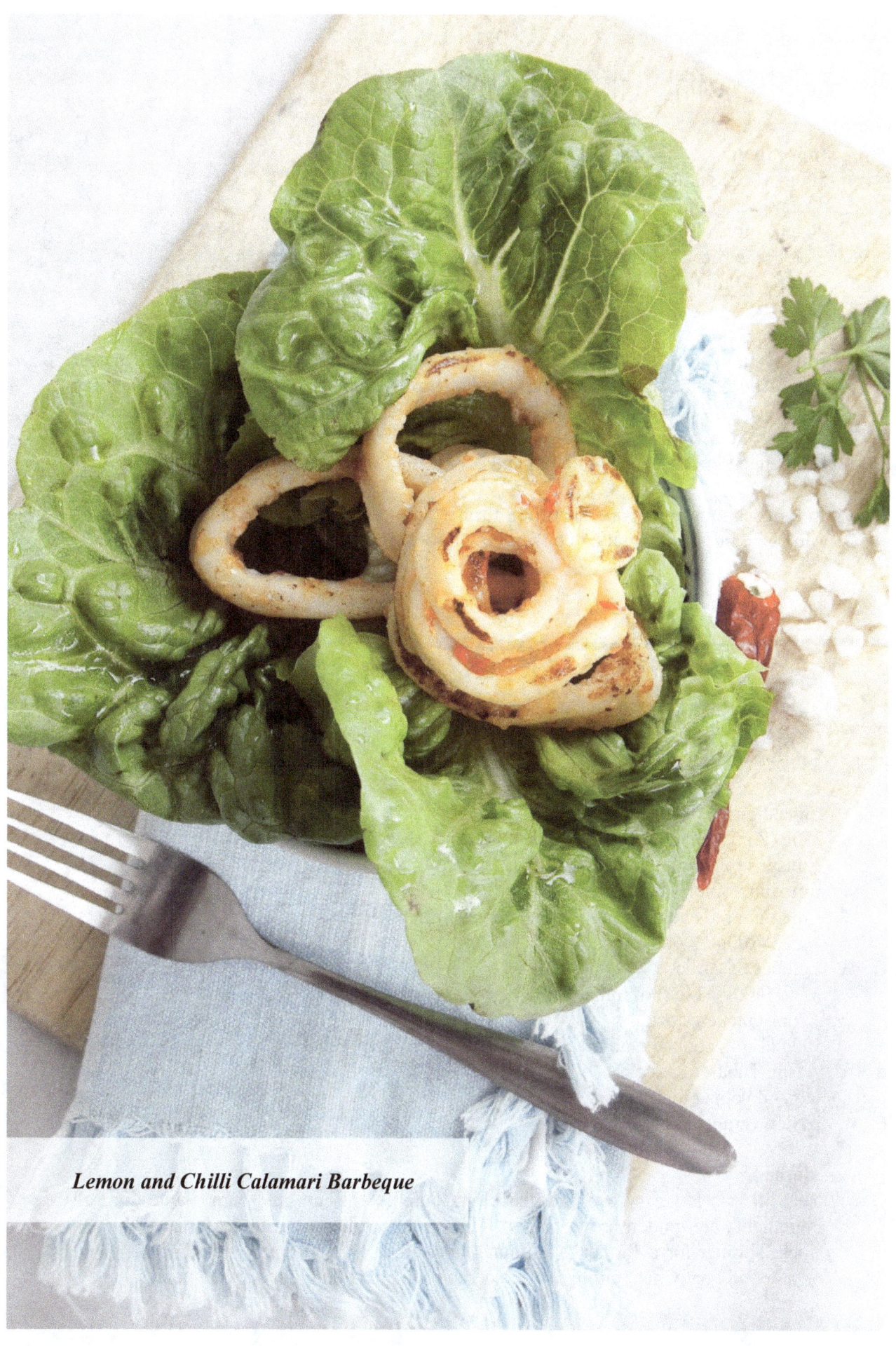
Lemon and Chilli Calamari Barbeque

SCALLOP AND CHERRY TOMATO SAUTÉ

Ingredients
500g (16oz) scallops
4 tspns corn flour
2 tspns olive oil
3 cloves garlic
⅔ cup (170ml / 5¾fl oz) white wine or chicken stock
salt and pepper
½ cup chopped basil
1 Aloe vera leaf
500g (18oz) cherry tomatoes

Method
Roll scallops in flour shaking excess off. Beat the oil in a frying pan over a medium heat. Add scallops and cook until golden brown. About 3 minutes. Using a holey spoon, scoop out into a bowl. Add minced garlic to the fry pan for 1 minute. Then add tomatoes and cook until they begin to collapse about 4 minutes. Add wine or stock, salt pepper and basil. Bring to boil and cook for a further minute.

Return scallops to pan and heat for a further minute turn off heat and mix the blended Aloe vera into the dish. It can be served with very thin noodles, or a light salad.

CRAB SAUTÉ

Ingredients
250g (8oz) zucchini cut into 1½cm (½") thick slices
2 tblspns olive oil
1 medium onion (diced)
1 medium red and green capsicum (pepper) finely chopped
¾ cup (100g / 3½oz) diced ham
2 cloves of garlic
1 can (400g / 14oz) of tomatoes
2 cups chicken stock
500g (18oz) cooked crab meat
¼ tspn Tabasco sauce
salt and pepper to tastes
1 Aloe vera leaf

Method
Heat oil in a large fry pan. Add zucchini, onion, capsicum and ham. Sauté until all ingredients are golden brown. About 10 minutes. Add garlic, tomatoes and chicken stock, simmer for a further 20 minutes uncovered. Stir in crab meat, Tabasco, salt, pepper and gently heat through. Take off the heat and add blended Aloe vera.

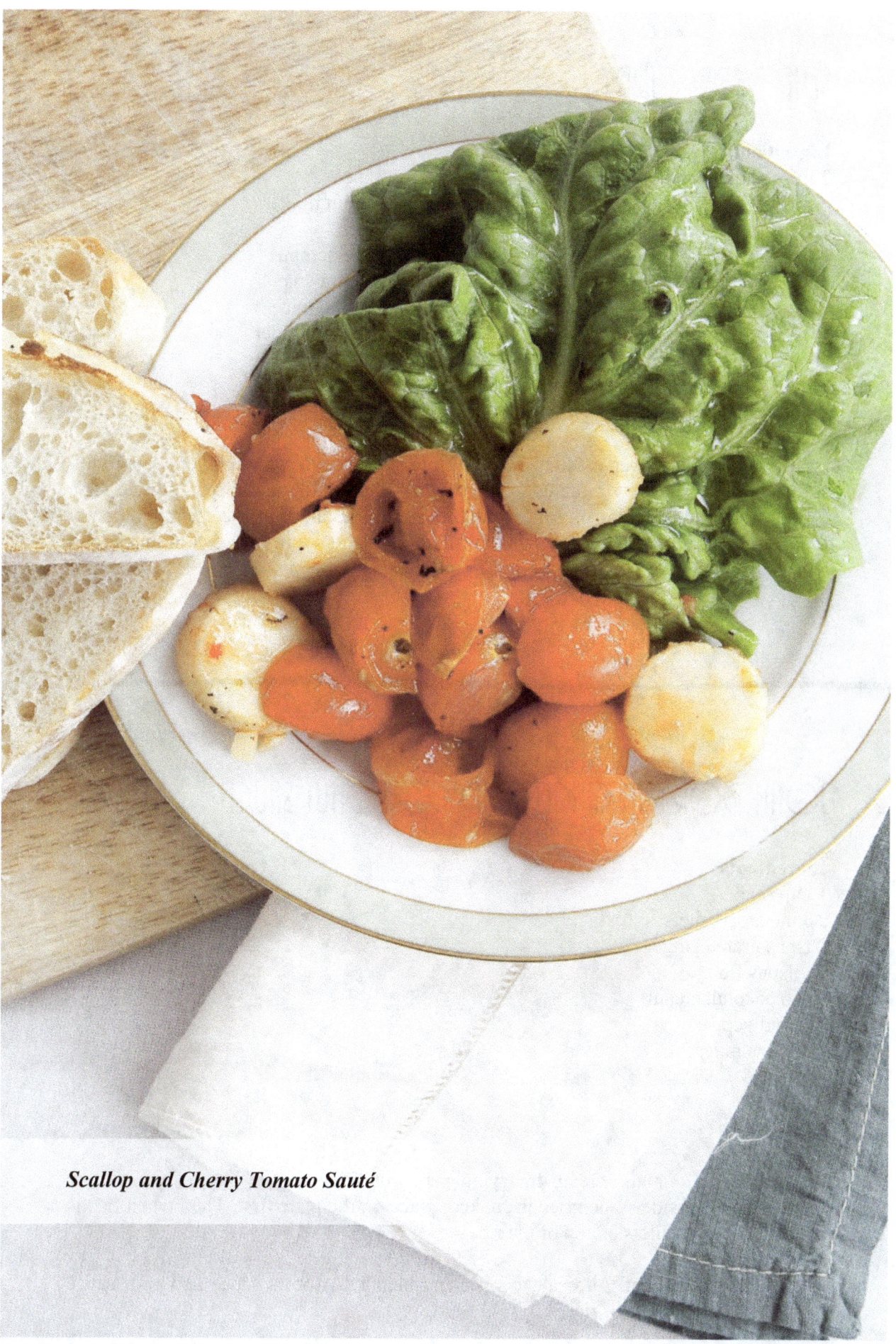

Scallop and Cherry Tomato Sauté

SEAFOOD CURRY

Ingredients

2 tblspns olive oil
6 spring onions
1 medium capsicum (pepper)
1 tblspn ginger
1½ tspns curry powder
¼ tspn chilli powder
¼ tspn Allspice
50g scallops
1 Aloe vera leaf
1 tblspn soy sauce
1 can light coconut milk
3 Roma tomatoes
50g (1¾oz) baby octopus
250g (9oz) med prawns
2 tblspns fresh lime juice
1 tblspn chopped coriander
250g (9oz) mussels
1 tspn cumin

Method

Heat oil in fry pan over medium heat add onions, capsicum and ginger. Sauté until softened, takes around 5 minutes. Add curry powder, chilli, and allspice. Sauté for a further 2 minutes. Stir in soy sauce, salt, coconut milk and tomatoes. Simmer gently for 15 minutes. Add fish and prawns to mixture simmer gently for 5-8 minutes until cooked. Then add coriander, lime juice and blended Aloe vera juice. Place the curry on a bed of freshly cooked rice.

JOHN DORY IN GINGER AND COCONUT SAUCE

Ingredients

1 cup rice
2 John Dory fillets
2 tspns grated ginger
2 tblspns flour
1 can coconut cream
salt and pepper
1 Aloe vera leaf

Method

Boil rice.

Place ginger, flour and cream in frying pan. Put fillets in the pan to cook a few minutes on each side. When rice is cooked, place on the plate first. Then when fish is cooked place the fillets on top of the rice.

Then turn off the heat. Add salt, pepper and blended Aloe to sauce and pour sauce over the fish on a plate of rice.

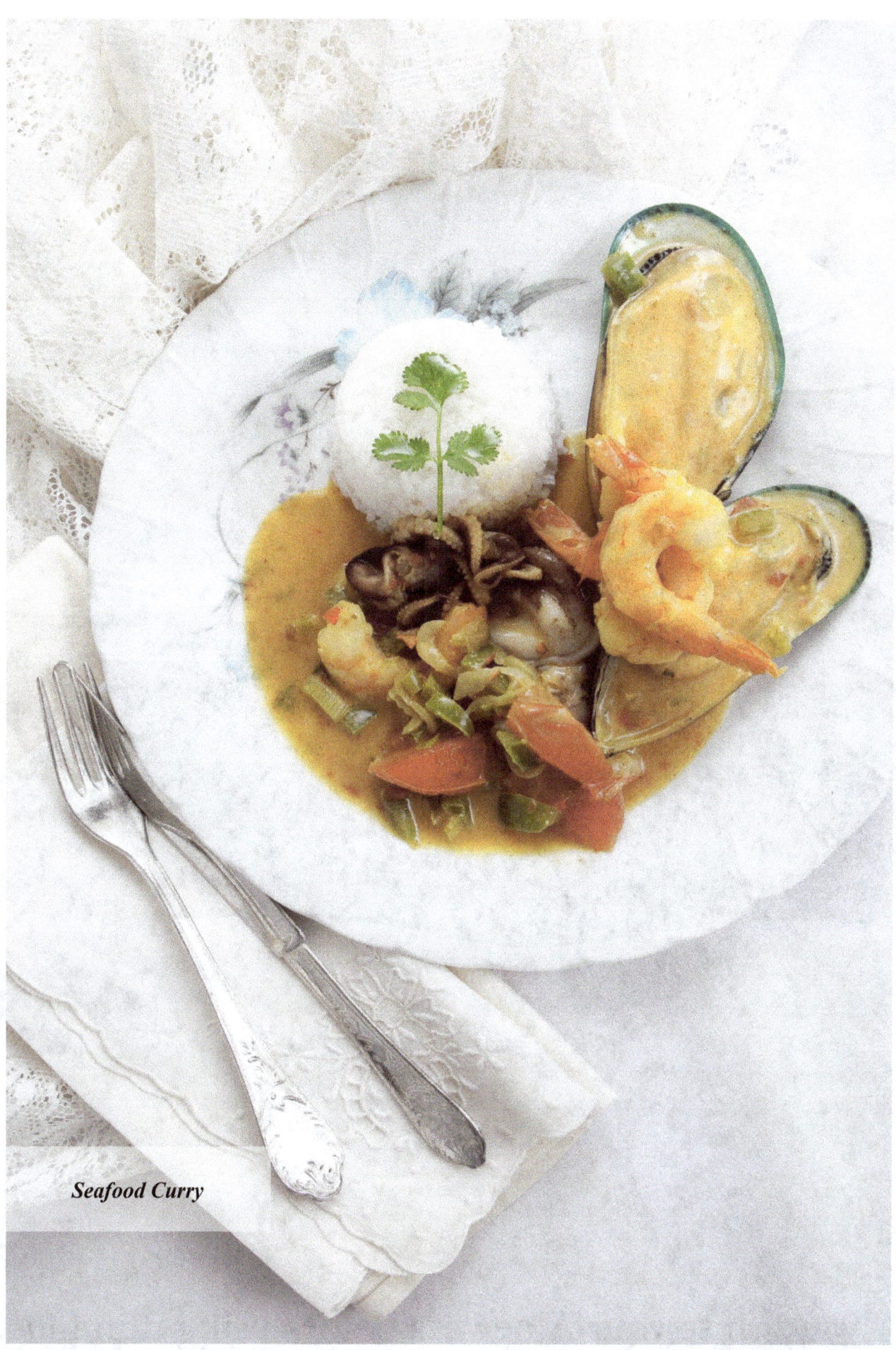
Seafood Curry

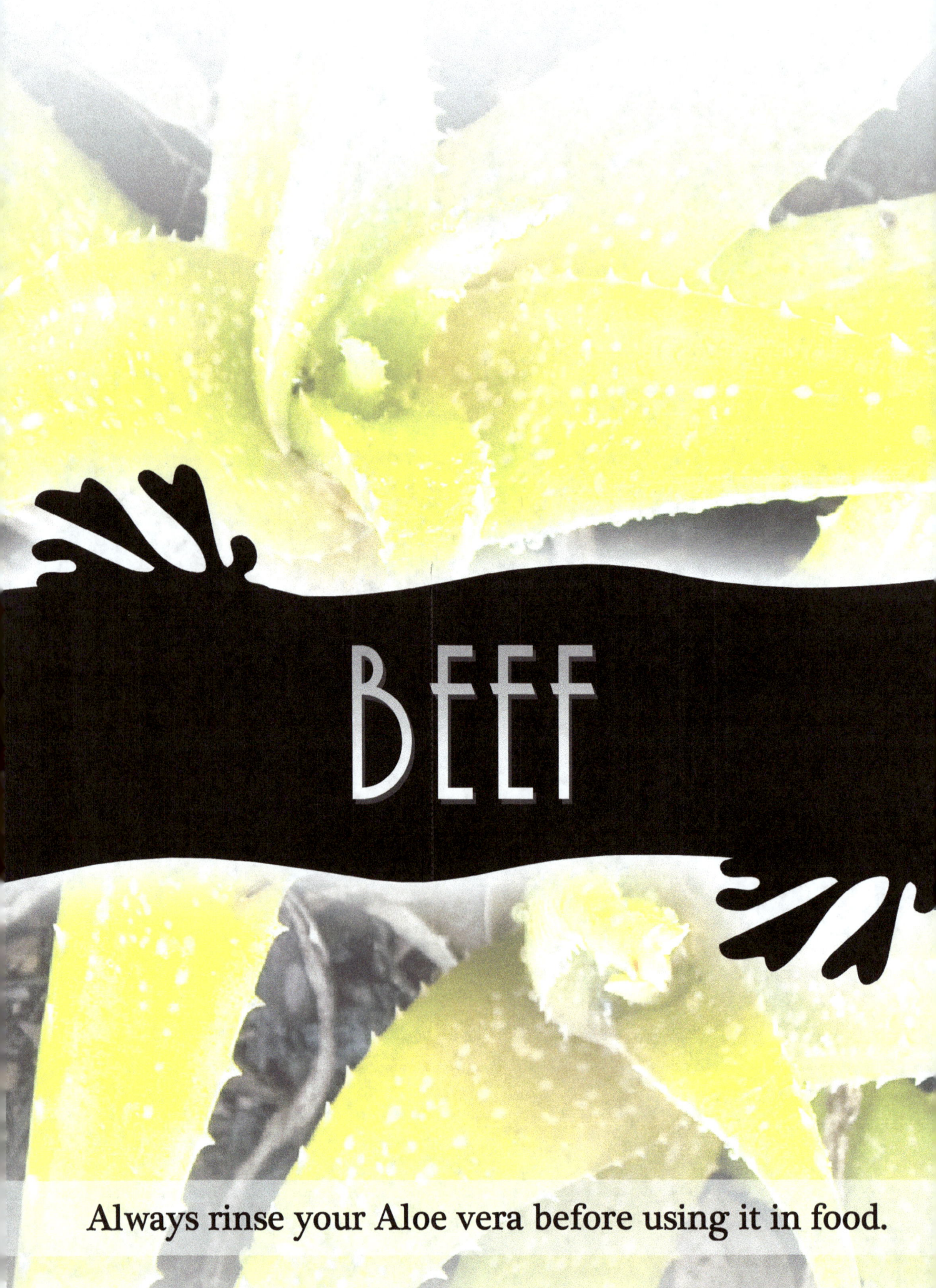

BEEF

Always rinse your Aloe vera before using it in food.

MOROCCAN BEEF

Ingredients
500g (18oz) lean beef
2 tblspns olive oil
2 cloves garlic
1 medium onion
½ cup slivered almonds
1 Aloe vera leaf
1 tspn ground cumin
1 tspn ground turmeric
1 can chopped tomatoes
60g (2oz) baby spinach
steamed rice (side dish)

Method
Cut beef into thin strips add oil and garlic and heat in fry pan/wok for 2 minutes. Put into a bowl and add oil onions, almonds, tomatoes and cook for a further 2 minutes return beef strips then add turmeric, cumin, spinach and add blended Aloe vera gel.

ORANGE AND BASIL VEAL BAKE

Ingredients
500g (18oz) lean beef
2 tblspns olive oil
1 tblspn plain flour
1 large onion
3 cloves garlic
salt and pepper
1 tin chopped tomatoes
250g (9oz) button mushrooms
1 tspn grated orange zest
½ cup orange juice
½ cup basil
1 Aloe vera leaf

Method
Slice onion and crush garlic and mushrooms, fry in oil with cubed veal that is slightly coated with flour for 2 minutes, place in casserole dish. Add tomatoes and juice add orange zest and juice salt and pepper to taste cover and cook for 45 minutes in oven at around 220°C (425°F). Stir in peas and basil and cook for a further 5 minutes then take out and add blended Aloe vera gel.

And serve with mashed potato or steamed rice.

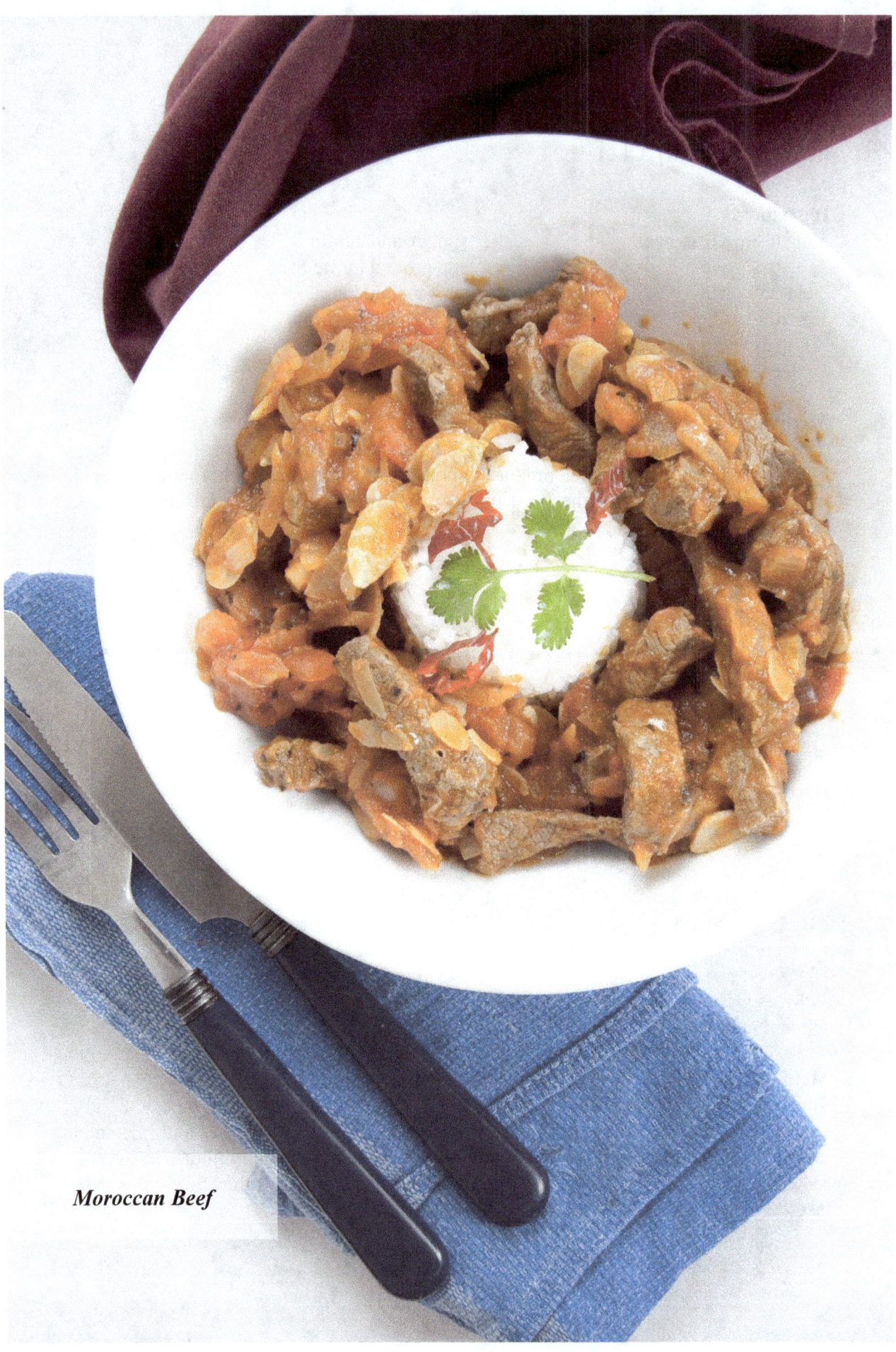

Moroccan Beef

VEAL IN ORANGE AND BASIL SAUCE

Ingredients

500g (18oz) lean beef
1 onion diced
2 cloves garlic
250g (9oz) mushrooms
3 fresh tomatoes
1 tspn orange zest

2 cups beef stock
1 tblspn basil
salt and pepper
1 cup frozen peas
2 tblspns plain flour
2 Aloe vera leaves

Method

Place a small amount of olive oil in the sauce pan, Slice thinly and lightly brown meat and then remove, add the diced onion, garlic, mushrooms, and tomatoes cook until softened. Beef stock, mixed Basil, salt and pepper. Cook for ten minutes and then add the cubed lean beef and cook for a further 1-2 minutes. Take off heat and add two tblspns of flour paste and the Aloe vera and serve.

BEEF/ROO STIR FRY

Ingredients

500g (18oz) lean beef
2 large carrots
2 stalks celery
1 large onion
2 cloves garlic (crushed)
2 Aloe vera leaves

2 tblspns BBQ sauce
salt and pepper
1 tblspn mixed herbs and rosemary
½ cup beef stock
1 yellow capsicum (pepper)

Method

Heat olive oil in fry pan, add finely chopped onions and diced carrots, stir for around 8 minutes, until veggies have softened a little. Then add celery, garlic, capsicum and stir for another 5-10 minutes. Slice beef/Roo into thin strips and put into pan. Add BBQ sauce, salt, pepper, herbs and beef stock. Cook for 2 more minutes. Take off heat and mix the Aloe vera juice into the meal just before serving.

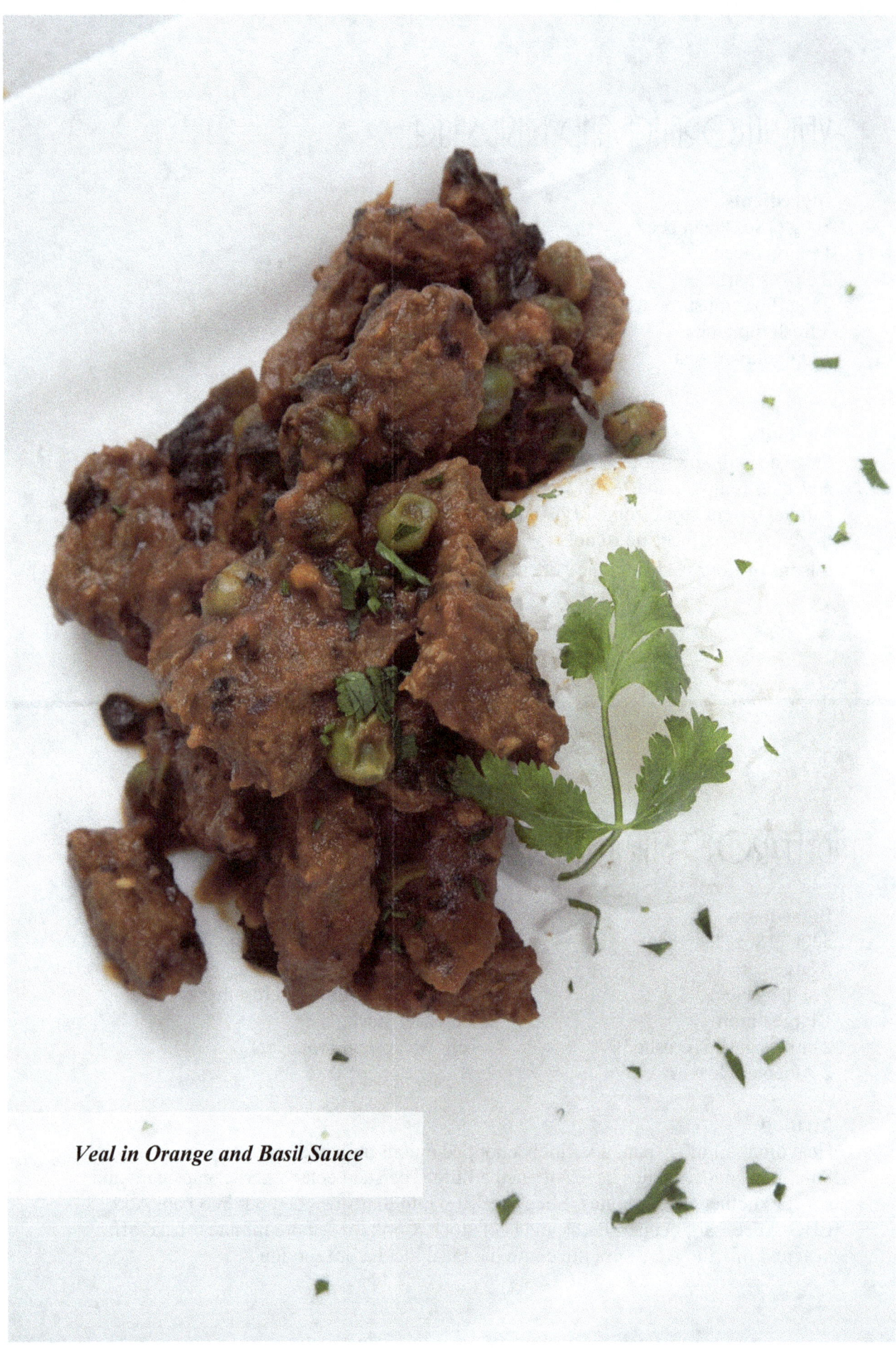

Veal in Orange and Basil Sauce

BEEF/ROO CURRY

Ingredients

500g (18oz) beef
2 tblspns olive oil
3 cloves garlic
1 red capsicum
salt and pepper to taste
steamed rice (side dish)
1 tblspn red curry paste
100g (3½oz) button mushrooms
1 tblspn fish sauce
1 can coconut milk
½ cup fresh coriander leaves
1 Aloe vera leaf

Method

Cut into meat into thin strips and mix into a fry pan/wok with oil and crushed garlic cook for 2 minutes then remove from heat. Add capsicum and sliced mushrooms with a drizzle of water and steam for 2 minutes, return beef/roo add curry paste, fish oil, coconut milk and coriander leaves, salt and pepper. Blend Aloe vera add once taken off the heat

---

BEEF AND VEGGIE SALAD

Ingredients

500g (18oz) lean beef (veal)
½ tspn of mixed herbs
salt and pepper to taste
5 flowers of cauliflower
3 broccoli flowers
250g (9oz) cherry tomatoes
3 tblspns of chives
2 tblspns olive oil
1 tblspn red wine vinegar
2 tblspns water
4 cups torn lettuce
2 Aloe vera leaves

Method

Season beef on both side with herbs, salt and pepper and put aside. Cook Cauliflower and beans for around ten minutes in boiling water. Drain. Put cauliflower beans chives, tomatoes and parsley in a large bowl. Grill steaks for a few minutes on both sides. Combine oil, vinegar mustard, two tblspns of water and Blended Aloe vera juice, season with salt and pepper. Place all in a screw top jar and shake well. Cut beef into strips and add to vegetables pour any juices that maybe on the plate into the jar of dressing stir and pour over the beef veggie salad.

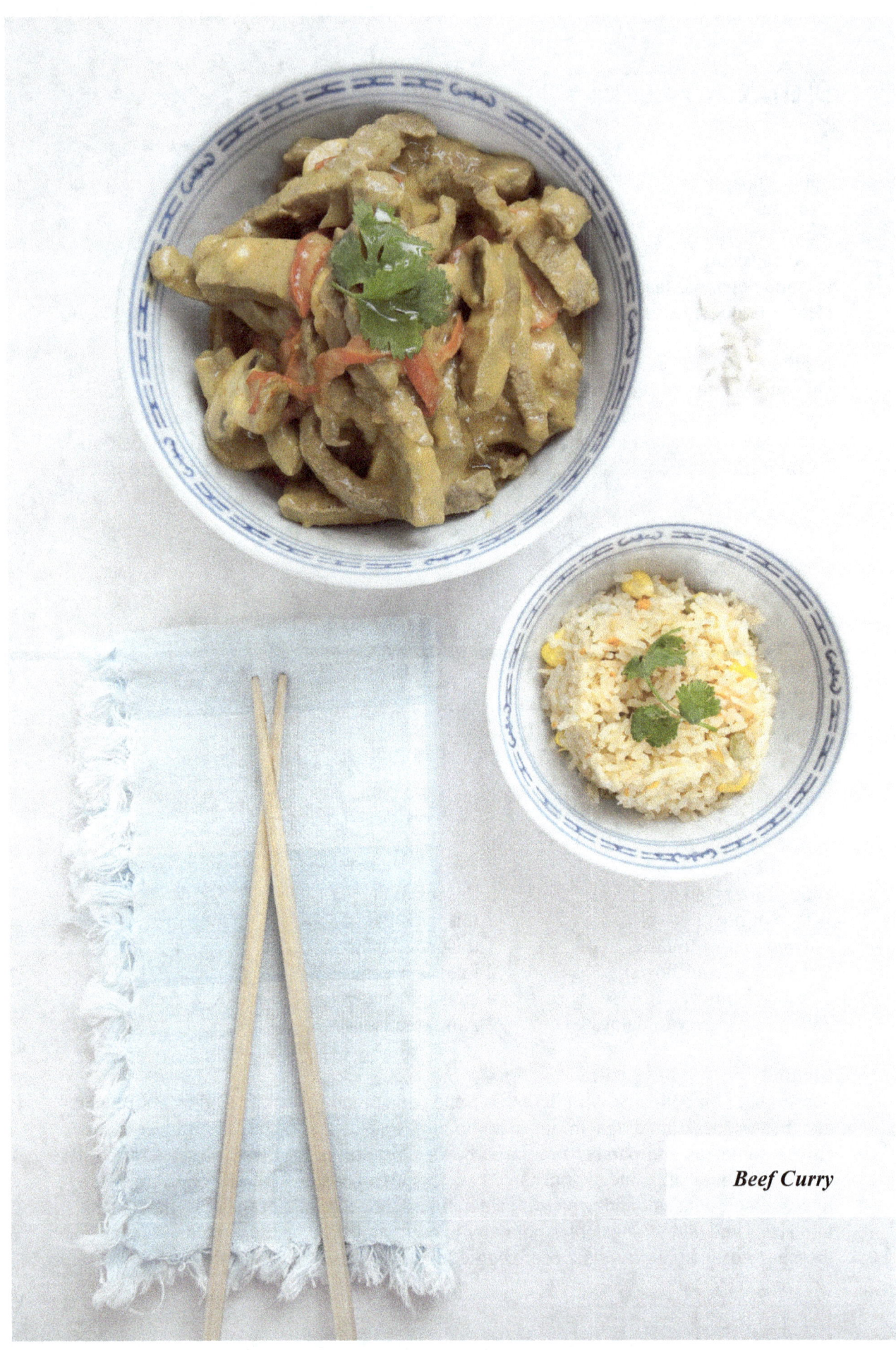

Beef Curry

THAI BEEF BURGER

Ingredients

2 tblspn tomato paste
½ cup (125ml / 4¼fl oz) lime juice
1½ tspns ground coriander
500g (18oz) lean sirloin beef
salt and pepper to taste
1 tspn chilli
2 Aloe vera leaves

3 cups shredded cabbage
2 large carrots
1 large capsicum
½ cup coriander
⅓ cup mint
4 bread rolls

Method

Blend the tomato paste half the lime juice and all the ground coriander and coat the beef well and leave to marinate for 30 minutes. Put the remain lime juice, chilli, Aloe vera, salt and pepper in a bowl add the cabbage, carrots, capsicum, coriander and mint, mix well and refrigerate. Cook steak lightly on a grill for a few minutes. The cut into thin strips and place into cut rolls with coleslaw salad.

BEEF AND VEGGIE WRAPS

Ingredients

500g (18oz) veal
1 onion
1 red, green and yellow capsicum
3 cloves of garlic
½ a cup of lime juice
2 tblspns olive oil
1 Aloe vera leaf, blended

2 tblspns balsamic vinegar
2 tspns cumin
salt and pepper
chilli to taste
flat bread
grated cheese

Methods

Chop garlic and chilli and put into a bowl, add lime juice, oil, vinegar, cumin, salt and pepper. Place steak onion and capsicum in a baking dish and pour the mixture over the steak, cover and refrigerate for 1 or 2 hours.

Preheat grill or barbeque. Cook steak for around 2-5 minutes on both sides and veggies. Let stand for 5 minutes. Then place blended Aloe vera into remaining marinate, mix well, and slice meat diagonally and pour remaining marinate over the steak and veggies and put the ingredients onto the wraps and sprinkle in the cheese.

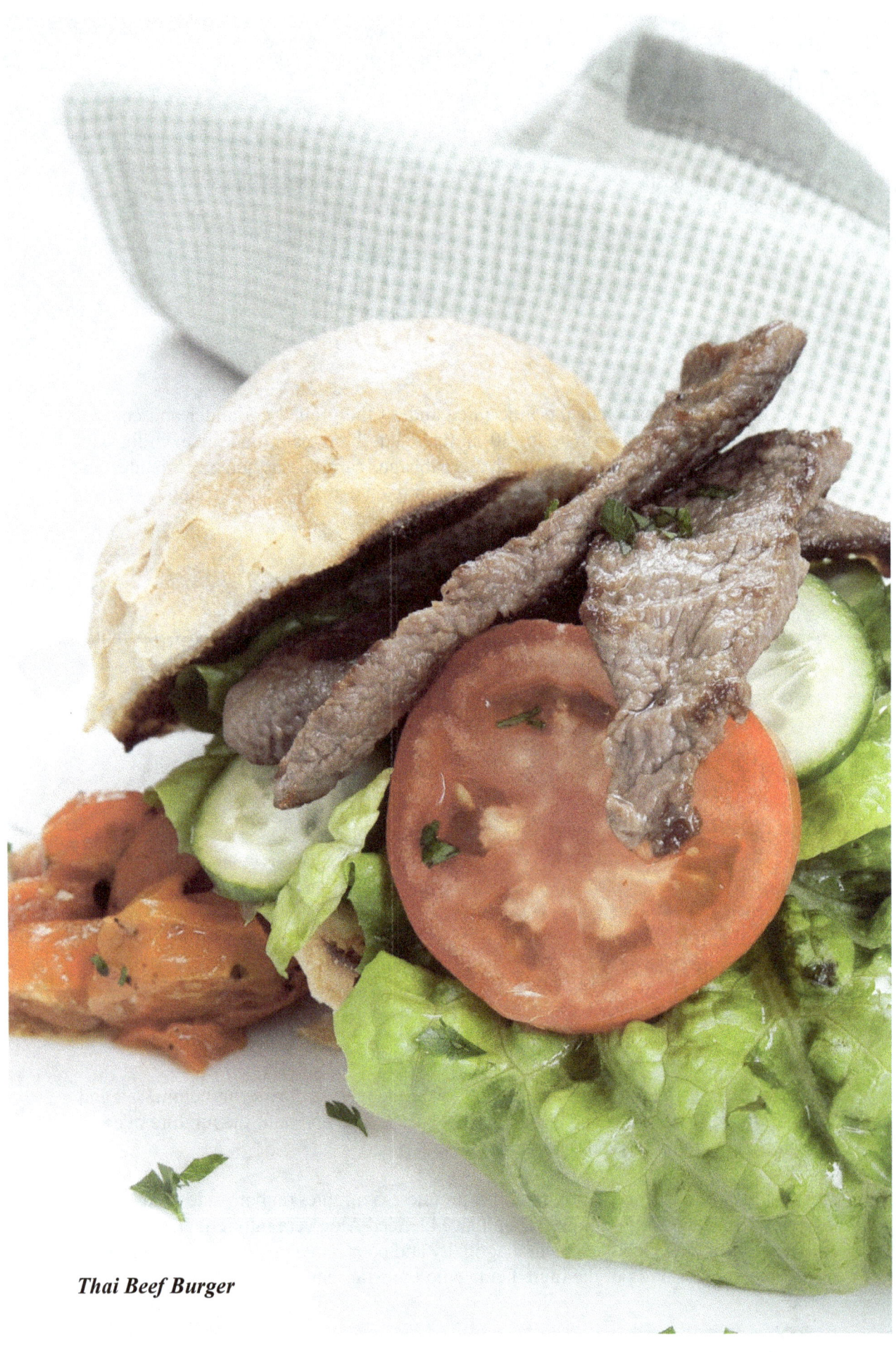

Thai Beef Burger

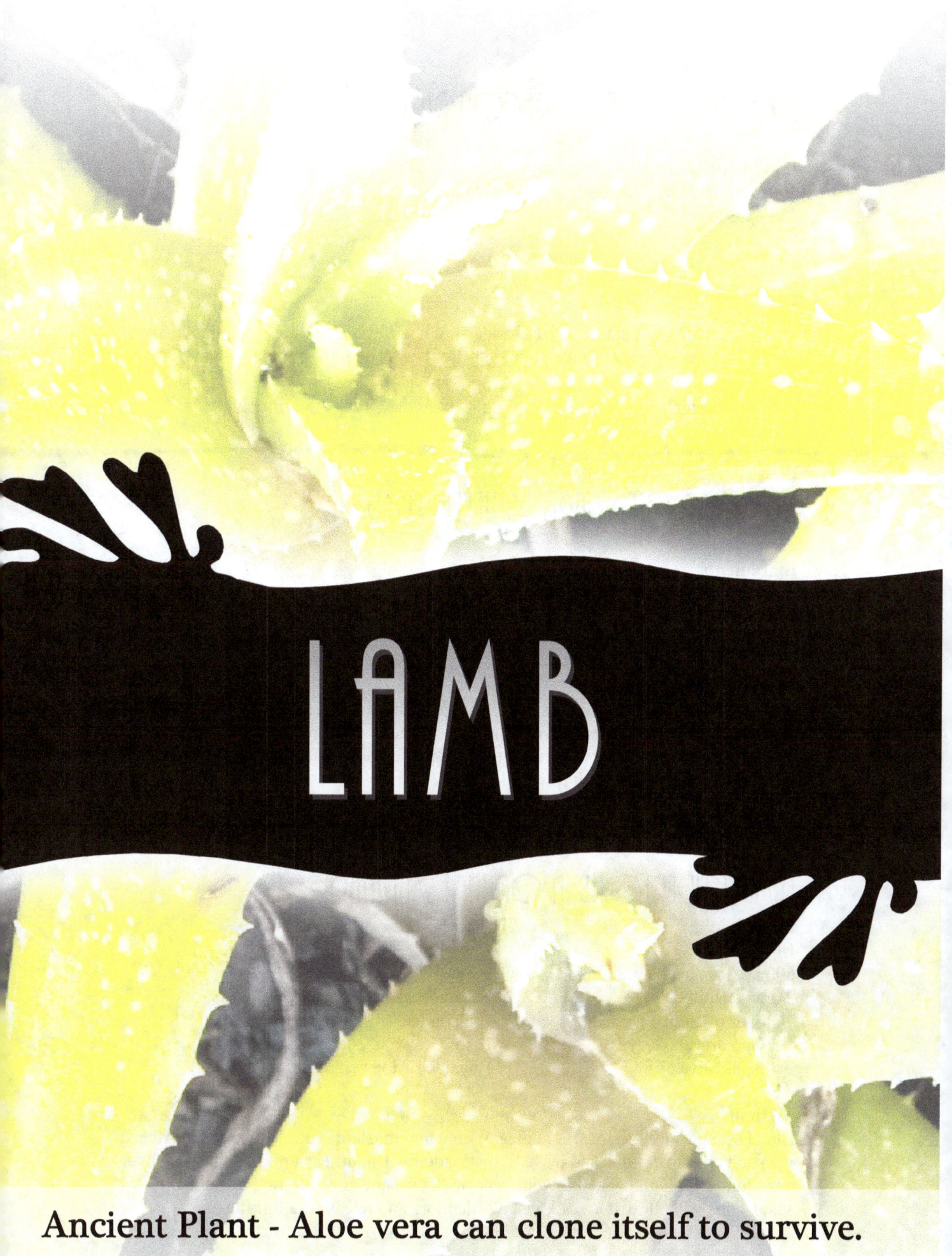

Ancient Plant - Aloe vera can clone itself to survive.

LAMB IN SAGE AND TARRAGON PASTE

Ingredients
600gms (21oz) lamb tenderloins
2 tblspns sage
½ cup basil
1 clove garlic
1 tblspn olive oil
1 tblspn tarragon leaves
1 Aloe vera leaf

Method
Blend sage, tarragon, garlic, oil and Aloe vera in a blender until it forms into a smooth paste. Smother over the steak well and grill or barbeque for 2 minutes or until you like the meet cooked.
Serve with salad.

ROSEMARY AND GARLIC STUFFED LAMB

Ingredients
600g (21oz) lamb steaks
2 tblspns olive oil
4 sprigs rosemary
3 cloves garlic
1 Aloe vera leaf

Method
Mix garlic and rosemary and blended Aloe vera juice together. Slice pockets into the steaks and place the mixture into the pockets. Baste in mixture and grill until cooked to your liking. Remember to take off the heat just before it is ready and let stand for a few minutes this will cook it to your liking.

LAMB TENDERLOINS IN ORANGE MARINADE

Ingredients
600g (21oz) lamb tenderloins
2 oranges juiced
2 cloves of garlic (crushed)
1 tblspn oregano leaves
2 tblspns olive oil
½ orange zest
1 tblspn balsamic vinegar
1 tspn brown mustard seed
1 blended Aloe vera leaf

Method
Blend orange juice, zest, garlic, vinegar, oregano, mustard seeds, and blended Aloe vera and pour over lamb and leave to marinade for 1 hour. Heat oil in frying pan over a medium heat until cooked to your taste and marinade after cooking and allow to stand - this will allow it to cook just a little more and release the full flavour.

Rosemary and garlic stuffed lamb

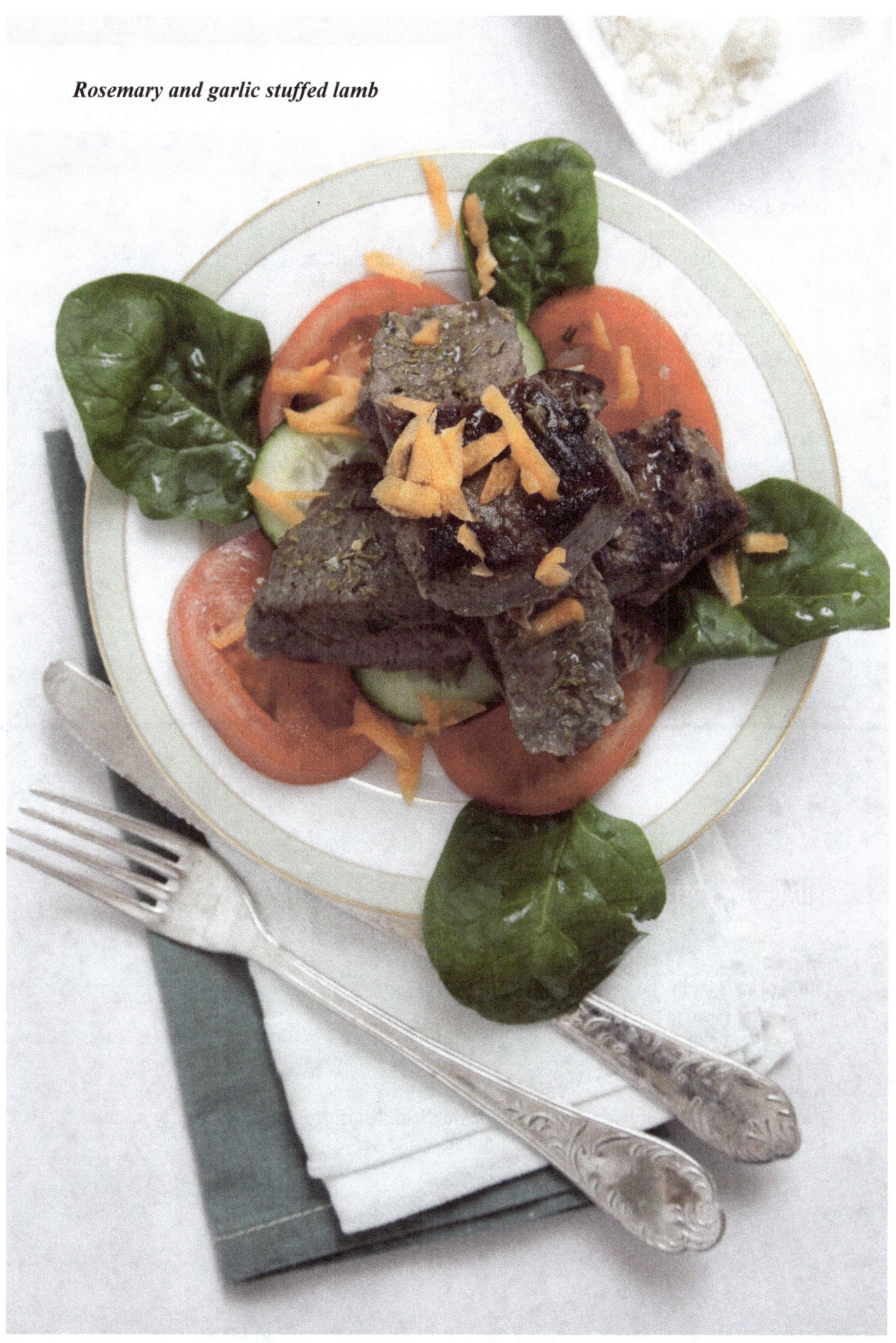

LAMB MEATBALLS

Ingredients
500g (18oz) lean minced lamb
1 egg lightly beaten
1 cup breadcrumbs
1 cup crushed Pine Nuts
salt and pepper
2 cloves garlic
2 Aloe vera leaves blended
1 tspn chilli powder
1 tspn rosemary
1 tspn ginger
1 tblspn olive oil
1 can chopped tomatoes

Method
Blend bread crumbs, salt, pepper, chilli powder, rosemary, ginger garlic and crushed pine nuts. Place into a large bowl with mince and egg and mix well, shape the mixture into small meat balls. Brown balls in fry pan once browned add tinned tomatoes cook for five minutes. Turn off the heat and add blended Aloe vera leaf and serve with spaghetti.

LAMB IN MINT SAUCE MARINADE

Ingredients
500g (18oz) lamb chops
fresh mint paste in a tube
1 Aloe vera leaf

Method
Baste chop with mint paste and blended Aloe leaf. Marinate for at least thirty minutes. Grill on the barbecue. Drizzle with mint sauce and serve.

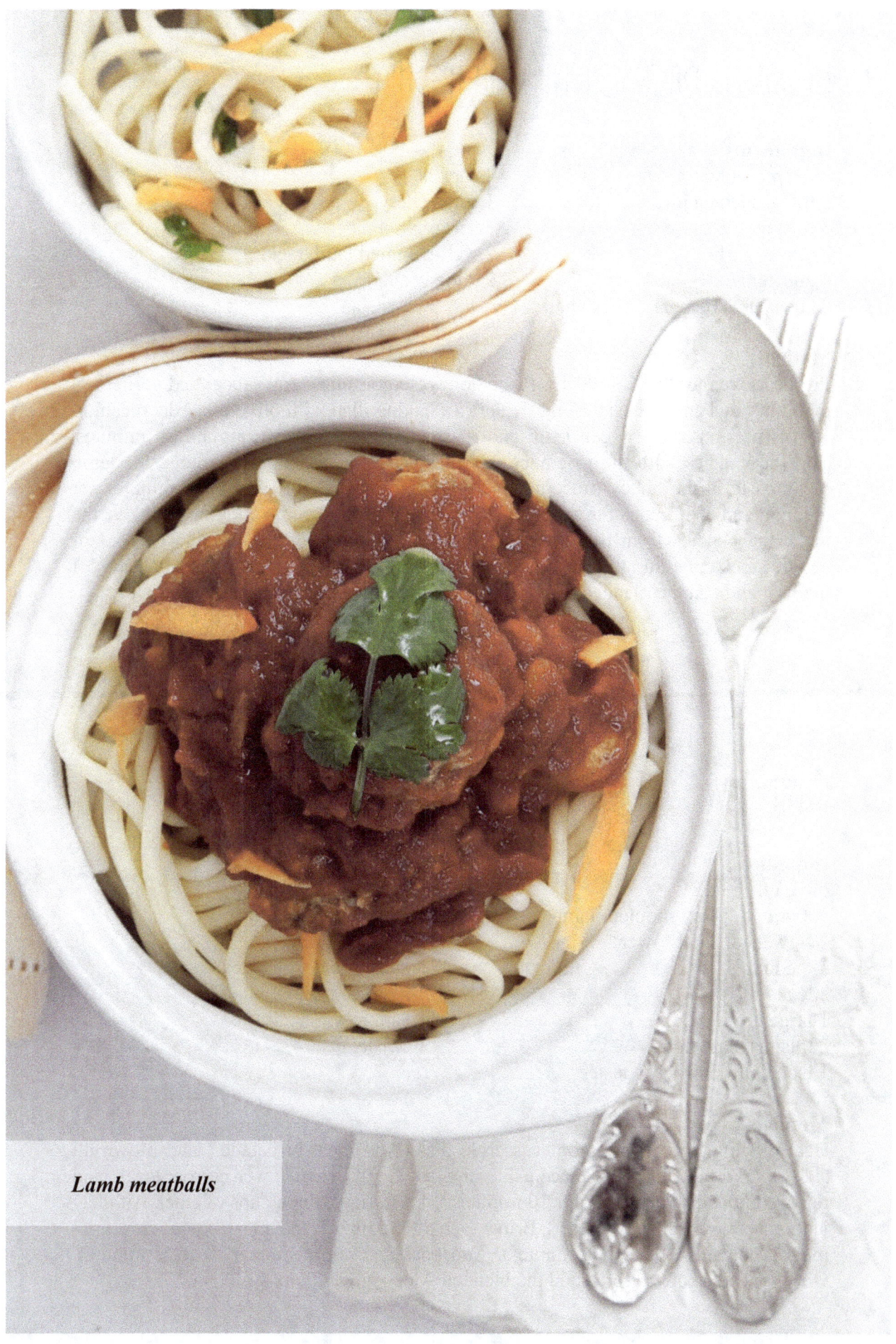

Lamb meatballs

ROASTED RACK OF LAMB IN HONEY

Ingredients
3 tblspns honey
3 tblspns lemon juice
3 tblspns soy sauce
2 cloves garlic
4 zucchini
2 capsicums (peppers) cut in half
4 carrots
1 stalk celery
6 sprigs rosemary
2 well-trimmed lamb racks
2 Aloe vera leaves

Method
Pre-heat oven to 200°C (400°F). Place honey, lemon juice, soy sauce, and garlic in a medium bowl and put aside. Lightly spray a baking dish with olive oil. Add zucchini, carrots parsnips, celery, capsicum and roast until golden brown around 20 minutes. Top the veggies with the rosemary and the pour over the stock. Arrange the lamb racks baste in the honey sauce and roast for 20 minutes for rare or 30 minutes for medium and 40 minutes for well done, continually basting while cooking. Remove the meat and veggies from the dish and put 3 table spoons of flour and 1 chicken or veggie stock cube into the pan and heat until thickened add water if needed. Take off the heat and add the blended Aloe vera juice to the sauce.

IRISH STEW

Ingredients
olive oil
500grams (18oz) shoulder lamb
4 flowers of cauliflower
3 medium carrots
2 leeks
1 large turnip
2 tblspns plain flour
1 tspn chilli powder to taste
1 cup of green peas
1 cup of frozen corn
salt and pepper
3 cups of chicken stock
1 Aloe vera leaf
1 tspn rosemary
1 bay leaf

Methods
Heat oil in a large flame-proof casserole dish. Add meat in batches, and brown all sides over a medium heat. Place aside in a bowl. Add cauliflower carrots leeks, and turnips to the dish and cook for 10 minutes. Mix in flour, three cups of stock with bay leaf, rosemary salt and pepper. Bring to boil. Simmer. Add meat, uncovered until meat is tendered (50 to 60 minutes). Add peas and corn. Simmer for five minutes. Once you are about to serve add the blended Aloe vera and mix well.

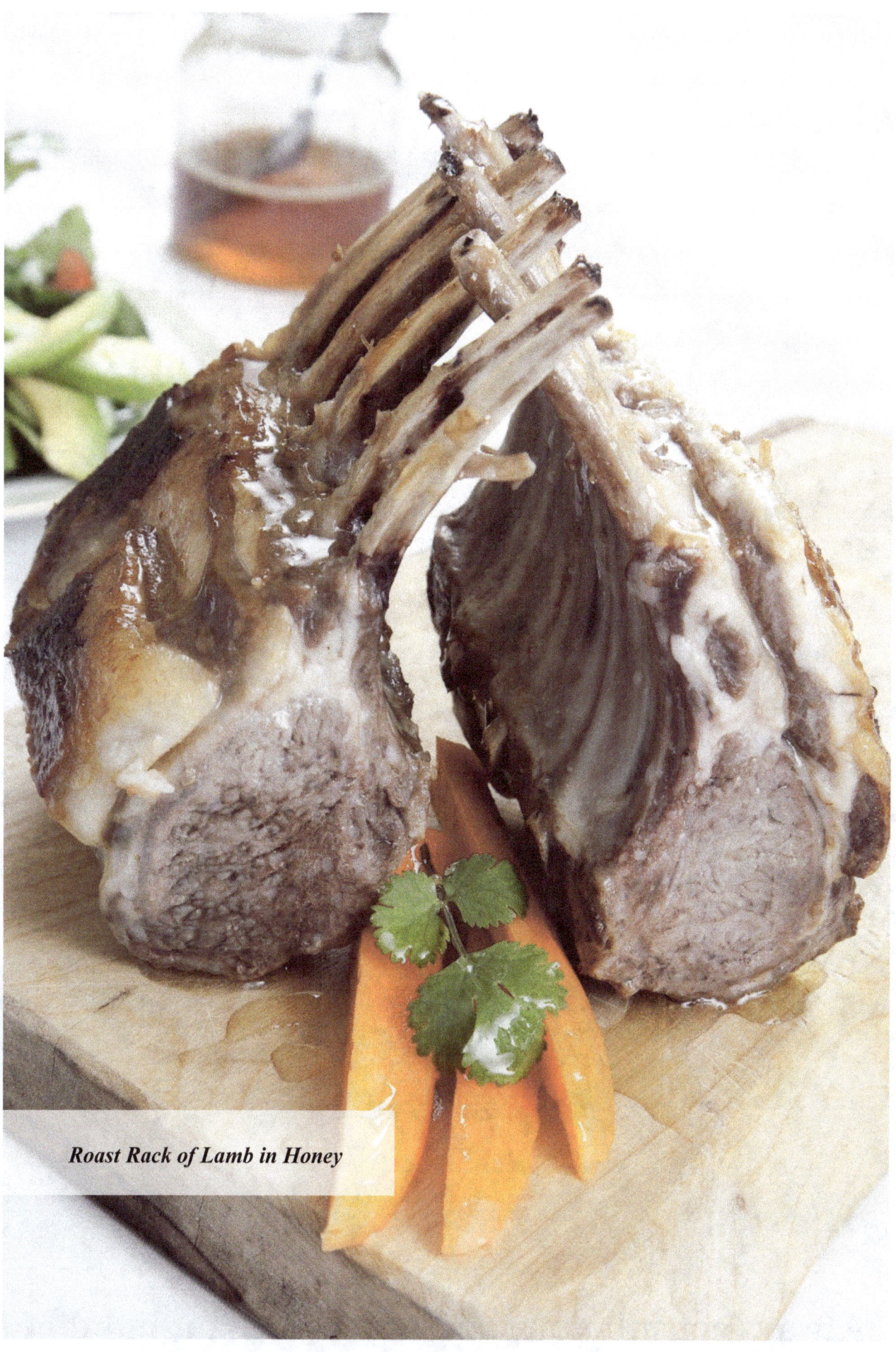

Roast Rack of Lamb in Honey

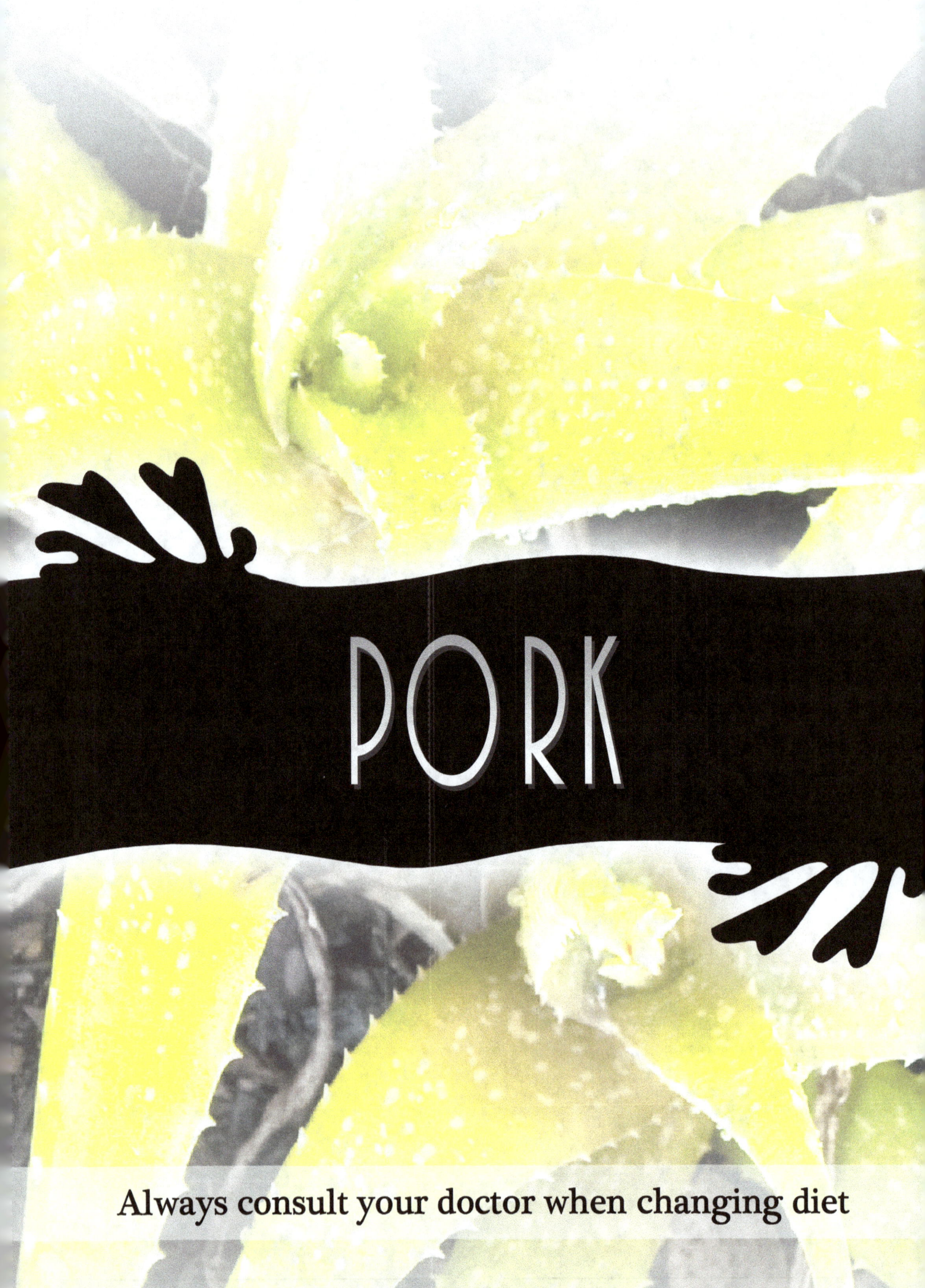

PORK AND BEAN CHILLI

Ingredients
750 grams (26½oz) pork shoulder, cut into small cubes
½ cup plain flour
2 tblspns olive oil
1 onion
1 medium capsicum
2 cans tomato
1 can five beans
1 cup chicken stock
1 tblspn chilli powder
salt and pepper
2 Aloe vera leaves
3 cloves garlic

Method
Roll pork in flour, shake off excess. Heat oil in a pan, on a high heat. In small batches add pork and brown all sides about 5 minutes. Lower heat to medium; add onion, capsicum, garlic and five beans. Cook until onion is golden and add meat and tomatoes, stock and chilli powder, salt and pepper. Simmer until meat is tender and sauce is thickened about 40 minutes. Take off the heat and add Aloe vera just before serving.

BOK CHOY STIR FRY PORK

Ingredients
2 cups chicken stock
2 tblspns soy sauce
1 tblspn corn flour
2 tblspn sesame seeds
salt and pepper to taste
500g (18oz) pork tenderloin cut into 3mm (⅛") thick slices
2 tblspns olive oil
5 cups bok choy
2 cloves garlic
pinch of tarragon and rosemary
1 Aloe vera leaf

Method
Blend together half the sherry and all the soy sauce, corn flour, herbs, sesame oil salt and pepper into a bowl. Smother the pork with marinate for around 15 minutes. Heat I tblspn of olive oil in a heavy pan or wok cook chopped bok choy for 2 minutes cover and cook a further 2 minutes transfer to plate remove liquid. Add remaining oil to pan Add garlic sauté until golden add pork mixture and stir fry meat until cooked 3-4 minutes Add bok choy and remaining cherry heat through. Take off heat and add blended Aloe vera and toss well serve immediately.

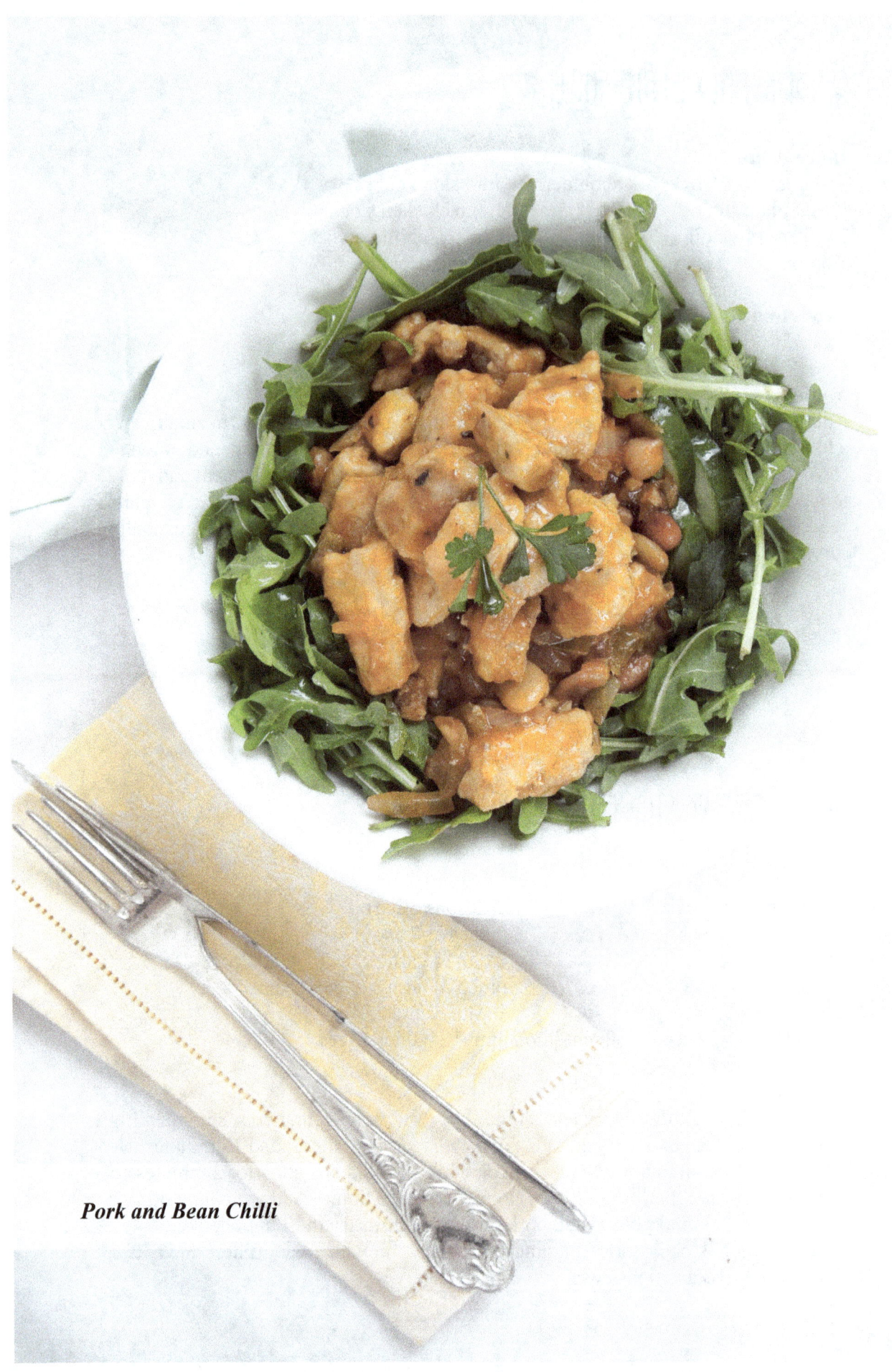

Pork and Bean Chilli

APPLE PORK STEAKS AND BEAN SALSA

Ingredients

8 lean pork steaks
2 tblspns olive oil
1 can three beans
½ cucumber
1 tspn Balsamic vinegar
1 Aloe vera leaf
2 tblspns apple sauce
1 tspn dried basil
1 purple onion
½ tomato diced
2 tblspns finely chopped parsley

Method

Mix apple sauce, dried basil and olive oil place steaks in fry pan and coat well with sauce. Cook for 2 minute each side.

Combine strained beans, onion, cucumber, tomato, parsley oil apple sauce and blended Aloe vera and balsamic vinegar. Place on plate beside the pork steaks.

STUFFED PORK WITH APPLE SAUCE

Ingredients

4 apples peeled and cored
1 cup water
2 cups bread crumbs
1 tblspn parsley
1 tblspn rosemary and sage
salt and pepper
600g (21oz) lean pork fillets
2 Aloe vera leaves

Method

Place cored and peeled apples in to a saucepan cover with water and bring to boil, reduce heat and cook for 20 minute or until soft. Remove 2 of the apples and slice and set aside. Blend the remaining 2 apples with chicken stock liquid to make a thick sauce. Place bread crumbs, parsley, sage, thyme, rosemary, salt and pepper into a food processor and blend until it is mixed thoroughly.

Cut the pork half way through along the top and stuff with the mixture. Place and divide the remaining apples in half and lay across the top of the pork and bake for 15-20 minutes in the oven at 220°C (425°F) oven. Once the pork is removed from the oven, blend the Aloe vera liquid into the apple sauce and mix well. Pour sauce over pork fillets.

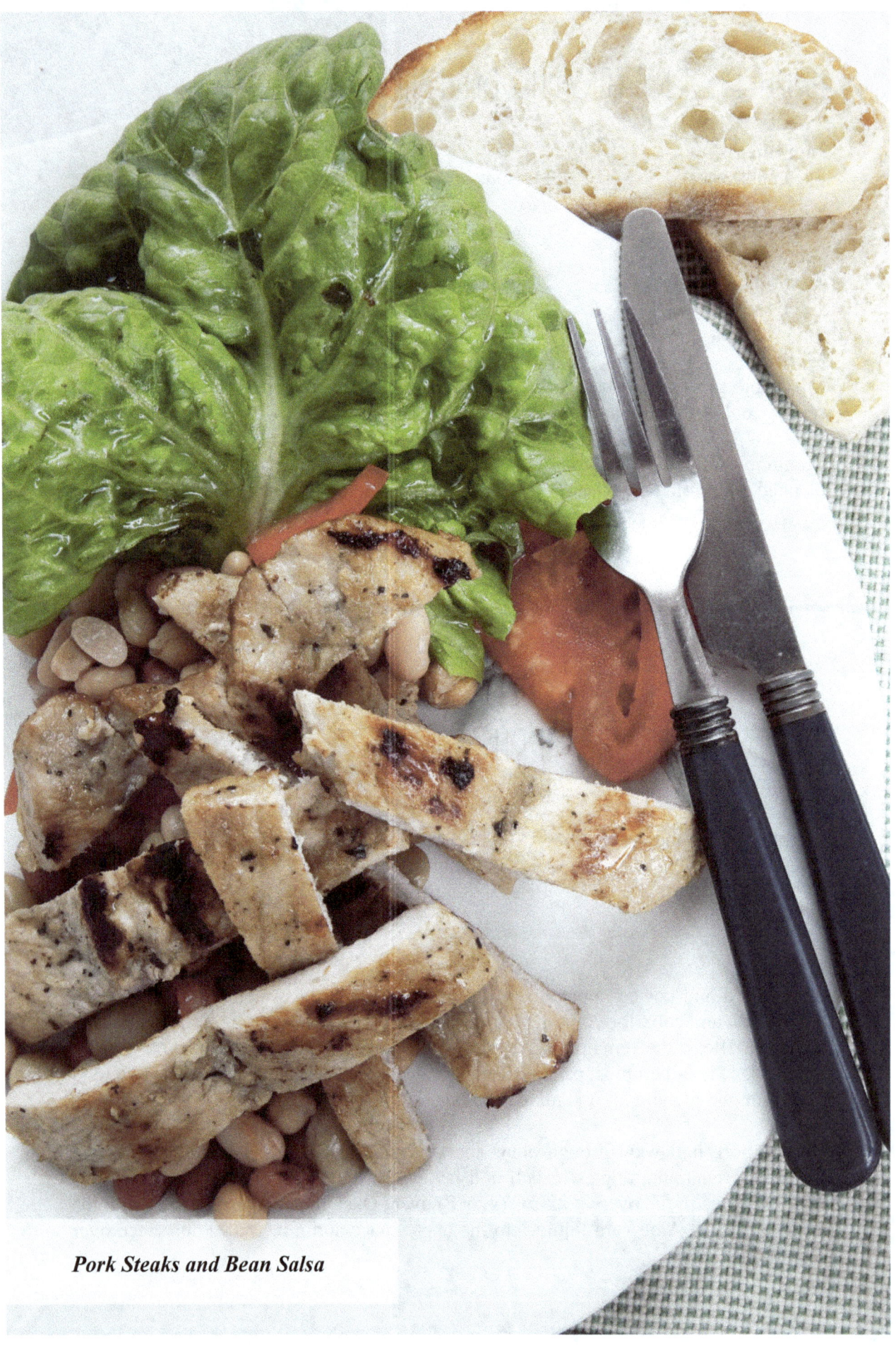

Pork Steaks and Bean Salsa

LEMON GRASS PORK SKEWERS

Ingredients
500g (18oz) lean pork
3 cloves garlic
1 tblspn soy sauce
salt and pepper to taste
1 Aloe vera leaf blended
2 tblspns of finely chopped lemon grass (white part only)
¼ cup coriander
2 tblspns BBQ sauce
3 different coloured capsicum (pepper)

Method
Combine crushed garlic, lemon grass, fresh coriander, soy sauce BBQ sauce and oil pepper and salt and blended Aloe vera leaf in a flat dish. Cube pork and soak in marinade for 30 minutes. Thread pork onto previously soaked skewers in between different coloured capsicums and cook in fry pan with olive oil for a few minutes on each side basting with marinade. Serve with a small bowl of chilli sauce if desired.

ROAST PORK WITH STUFFED APPLE AND ROSEMARY

Ingredients
1 pork leg roast
2 apples (thin pieces)
2 apples (finely chopped)
1 Aloe vera leaf blended
rosemary
2 tblspns honey
cinnamon

Method
Cut slits into the pork all over and place pieces of apple into them, then sprinkle with rosemary generously and roast for one to two hours depending on the size of the roast.

Peel, core and slice the apples, then place into a glass bowl with honey, and microwave for ten minutes. Scoop apple pieces into blending jug, add sugar, vanilla and Aloe vera gel. Blend until smooth.

Serve with roast veggies or salad.

Lemon Grass Pork Skewers

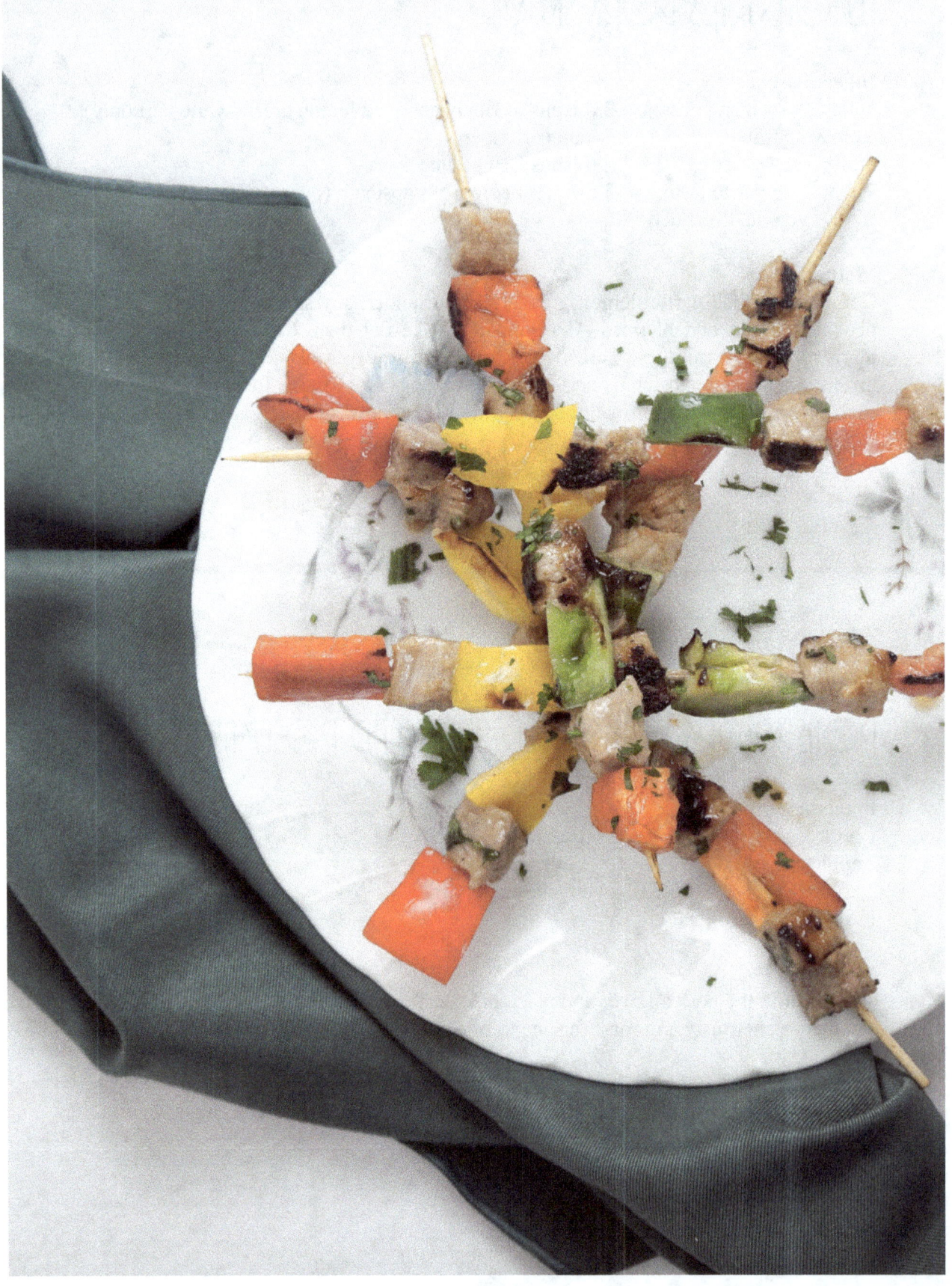

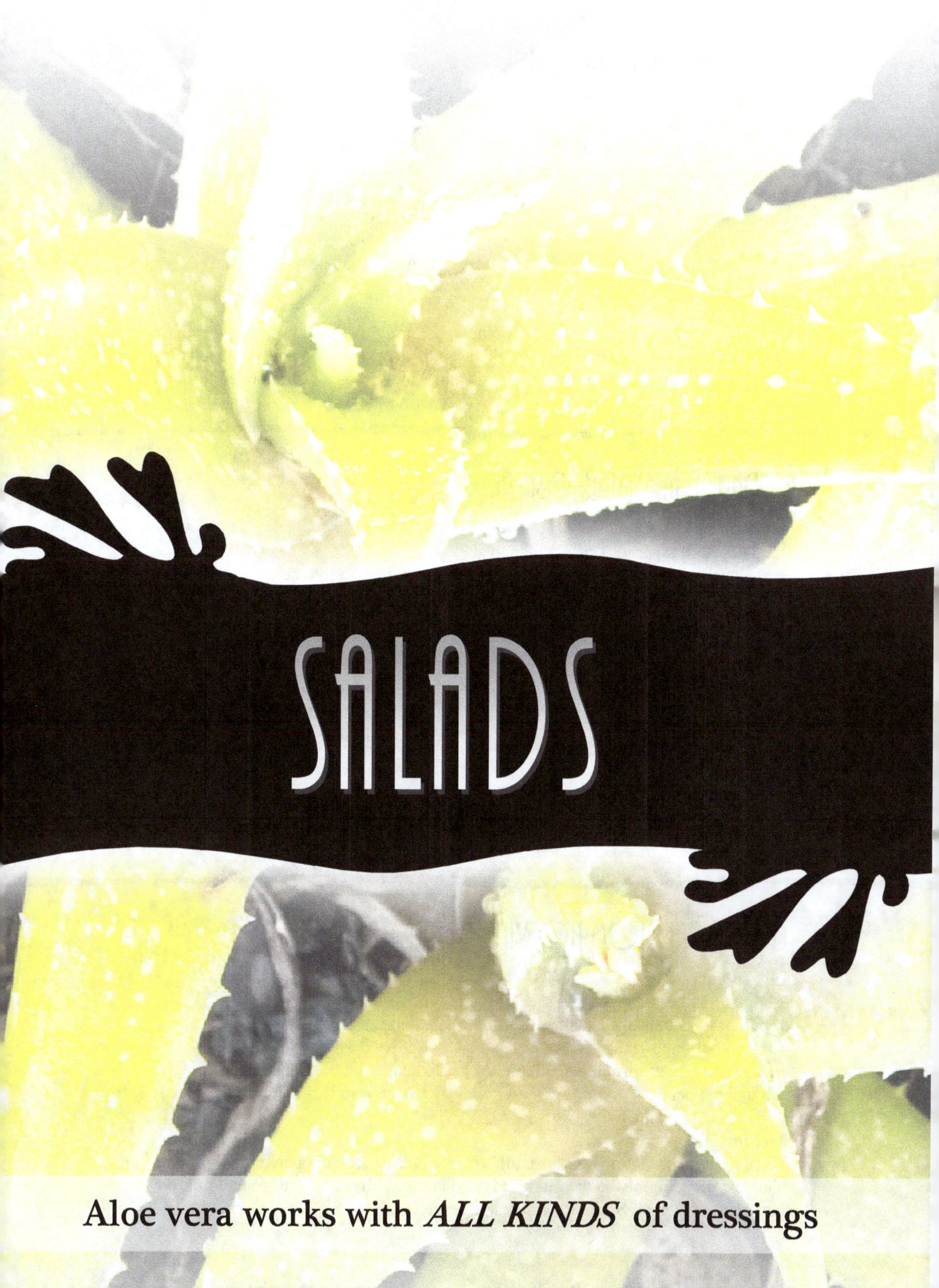

SALADS

Aloe vera works with *ALL KINDS* of dressings

CITRUS AND PINE NUT SALAD

Ingredients
2 oranges, peeled and segmented
200g (7oz) green capsicum
200g (7oz) snow peas
1 lettuce
1 cucumber
salt and pepper
¼ cup olive oil

Salsa
4 tblspns red capsicum
2 tblspns coriander
2 shallots
1 tblspn ginger
150g (5oz) pine nuts
1 lemon juiced
2 Aloe vera leaves

Method
Mix all the salad ingredients after slicing and lightly toss - add salt, pepper and olive oil. Then place chopped salsa ingredients into another bowl and mix well together with a stick blender, make sure the lemon and Aloe vera are well blended through.

ORANGE AND SESAME SALAD

Ingredients
350g (12¼oz) asparagus spears blanched
  (blanch: plunge into boiling water for one minute then into cold water to refresh)
2 Lebanese cucumbers
200g (7oz) green capsicum
2 spring onions
½ Spanish onion
3 oranges
1 lettuce
1 tblspn sesame seeds

Dressing
2 tblspns sesame oil
2 tblspns ginger
1 clove garlic
zest and juice of ½ orange
1 Aloe vera leaf blended

Method
Chop up all the salad ingredients and place into a bowl. Blend all the dressing ingredients and also mix well. Drizzle dressing over salad and serve

LETTUCE AND TOMATO VINAIGRETTE

Ingredients
2 large tomatoes chopped and seeded
½ cup of loosely packed basil leaves
1 tblspn balsamic vinegar
1 large cos lettuce torn into small pieces
salt and pepper

2 tblspns tomato sauce
2 tblspns olive oil
1 clove garlic
¼ cup crumbled feta cheese
1 Aloe vera leaf blended

Method
Place tomato, basil, tomato sauce, oil, vinegar, garlic, salt, pepper, and Aloe juice into blender. Blend lightly so the mixture is still chunky. Break up lettuce and mix the vinaigrette together. Sprinkle on feta and serve.

Orange and Sesame Salad

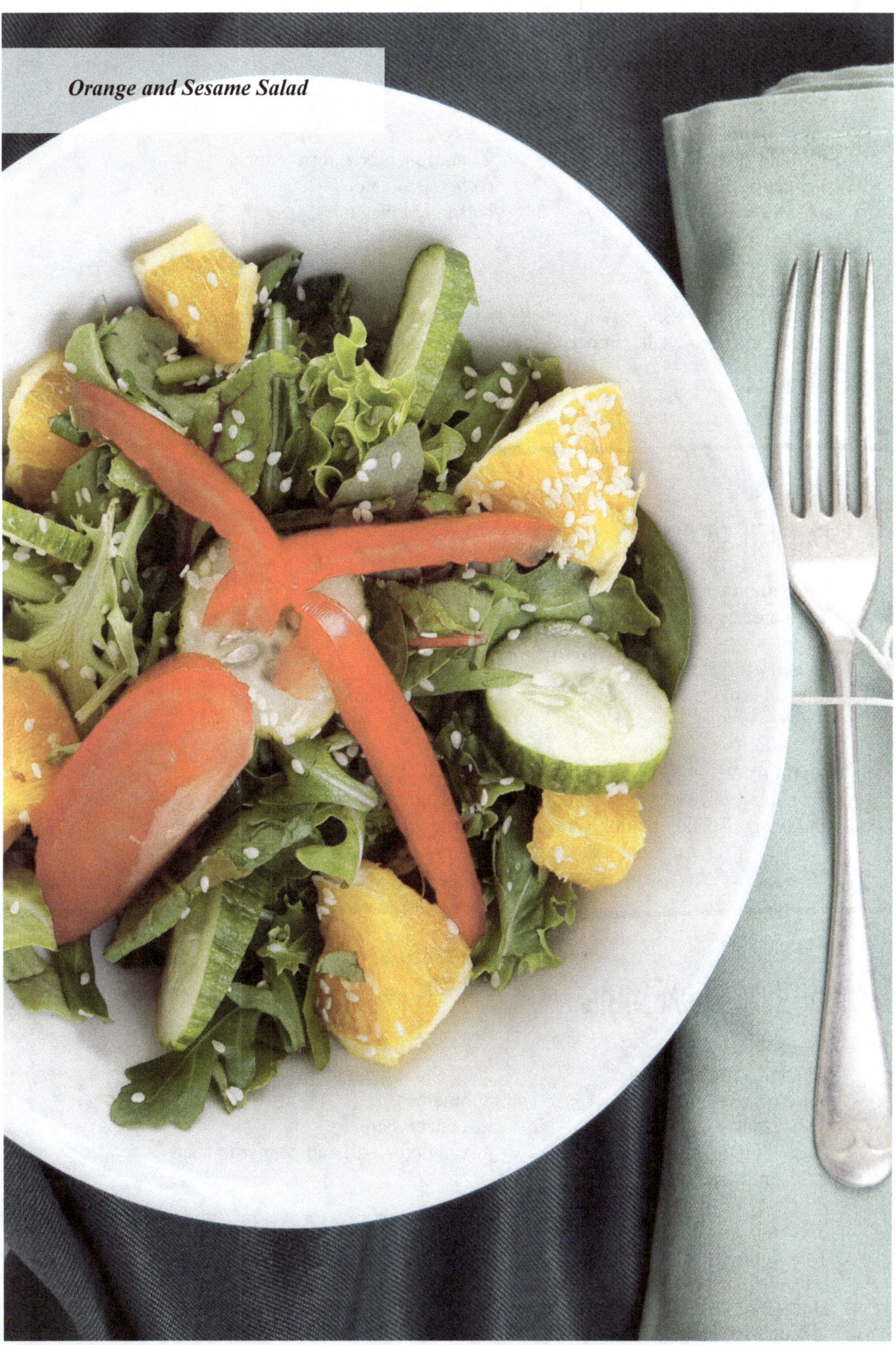

EGG SALAD

Ingredients
4 boiled eggs
3 slices of tasty cheese
mixed herbs salt and pepper
1 Aloe vera leaf
2 handfuls mixed torn lettuce
6 cherry tomatoes
balsamic vinegar

Method
Boil eggs remove shells, cut and add to torn lettuce, chop cherry tomatoes cube cheese add herbs, salt, pepper. Blend Aloe vera and balsamic vinegar and drizzle over salad.

RADISH SALAD

Ingredients
3-4 handfuls of mixed lettuce
2 apples
6 cherry tomatoes
mixed herbs, salt and pepper
1 Aloe vera leaf blended
4-6 radishes
1 cucumber
1 purple onion
2 tspns of sesame oil
balsamic vinegar

Method
Tear salad, slice radishes, apples, cucumber and onion. Chop tomatoes add herbs salt and pepper Blend oil Aloe vera and Balsamic vinegar and drizzle over the salad.

MUSHROOM SALAD

Ingredients
2 handfuls mixed lettuce
1 carrot
3 slices tasty cheese
toasted pumpkin seeds
2 tblspns sesame oil
250g (9oz) mushrooms
2 tomatoes
½ a cucumber
mixed herbs, salt and pepper to taste

Method
Tear up lettuce, clean and thinly slice mushrooms, cucumber grate carrot, cube tomatoes and cheese. Toast pumpkin seeds on a try in the oven for a few minutes. Once cooled add to salad also add herbs, salt and pepper. Blend Aloe vera and oil and drizzle over the salad.

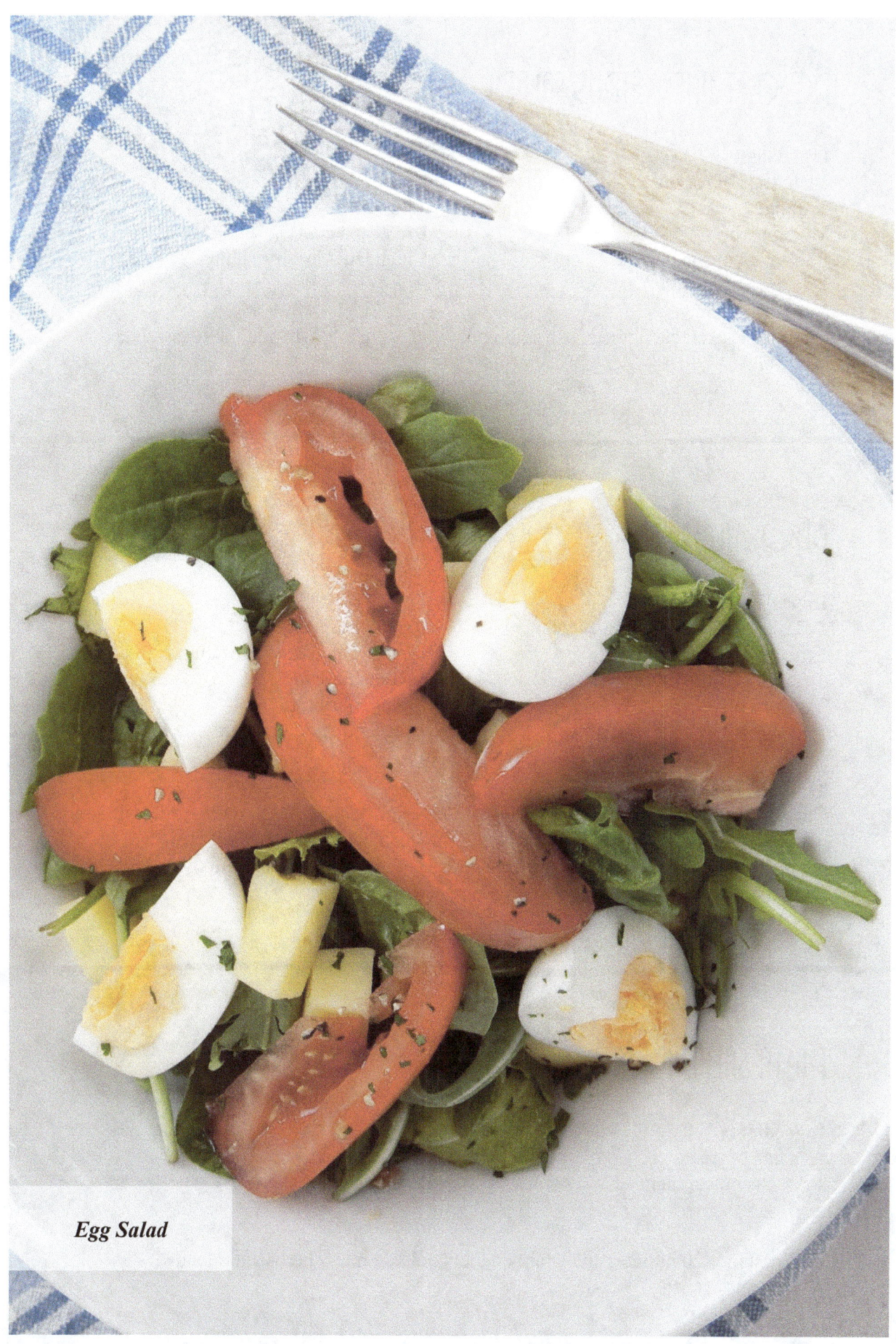
Egg Salad

ROCKET AND CITRUS SALAD

Ingredients

2 handfuls of rocket
2 oranges
Mixed herbs
Balsamic vinegar
1 tblspn sesame oil
1 cucumber
2 tomatoes
1 red capsicum
1 blended Aloe vera leaf

Method

Combine rocket, cucumbers, capsicum and oranges in a bowl. Add the dressing and mix well.

BBQ SALAD MIX

Ingredients

1 (350g / 12¼oz) medium eggplant
1 medium zucchini
2 cloves garlic crushed
2 tblspns olive oil
1½ tblspns balsamic vinegar
1 small bulb fennel
1 yellow and 1 red capsicum
3 Roma tomatoes
½ tspn marjoram
1 blended Aloe vera leaf

Method

Cut all veggies lengthways and spray with olive oil then sprinkle with garlic salt and pepper and place on the grill or barbeque. As each cooks place into a bowl and once all is finished put the marjoram vinegar and Aloe into the bowl and mix well and then serve immediately.

PASTA SALAD

Ingredients

½ a bag of pasta
1 Aloe vera leaf blended
Light mayonnaise
Mixed herbs

Method

Boil pasta for 20 minutes and strain and let cool add mayo herbs and blended Aloe vera.

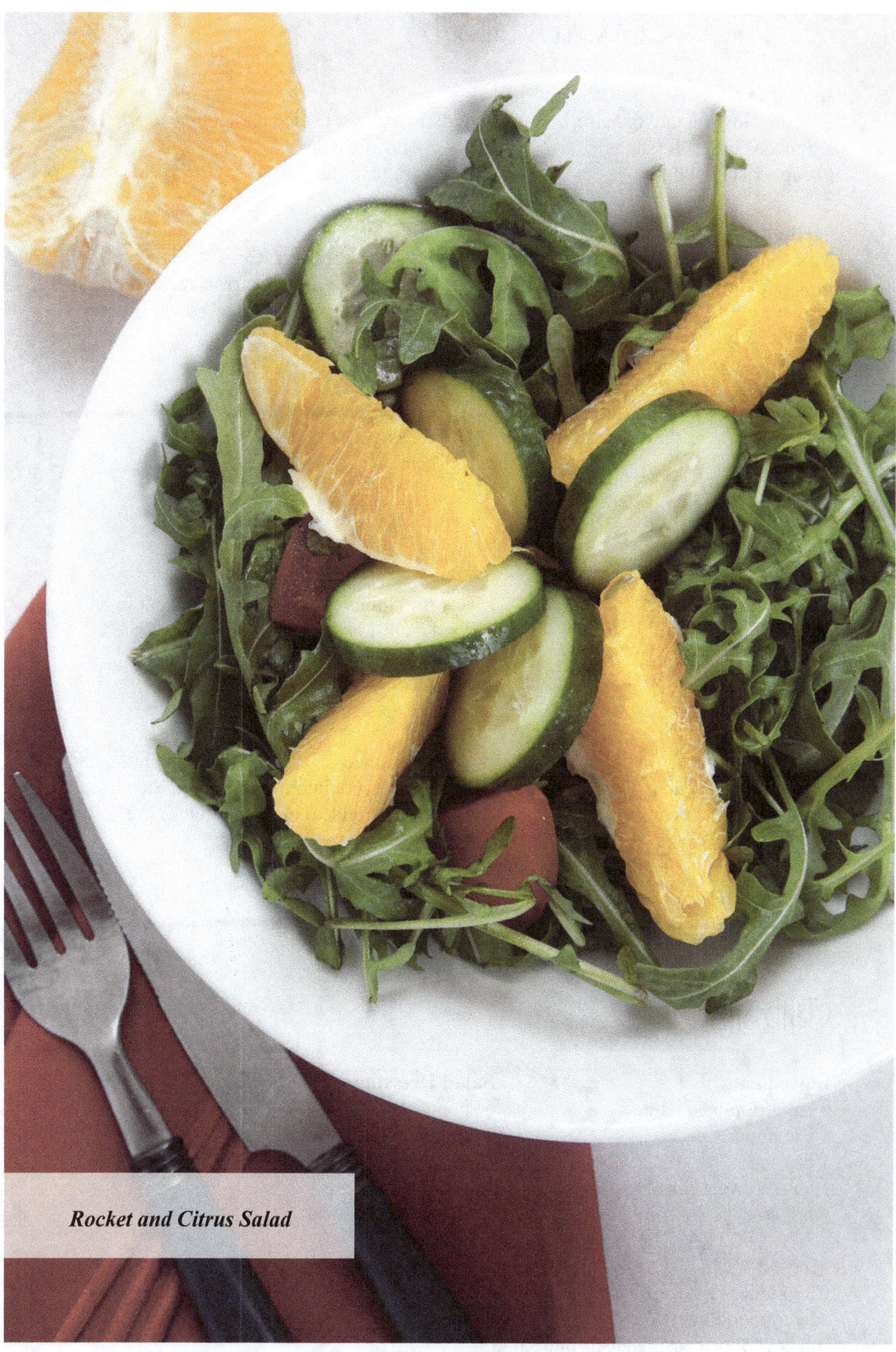

Rocket and Citrus Salad

ALMOND-BROCCOLI COLESLAW

Ingredients
3 tblspns low-fat mayonnaise
2 bunches broccoli (stems)
¼ cup roast almonds

2 medium carrots, peeled and grated
finely chopped parsley
1 Aloe vera leaf blended

Method
Mix the mayonnaise and Aloe together to make the dressing. Cut off the florets of broccoli and save for another meal, grate the stem. Add grated carrot, roast almonds in oven until golden and then add, parsley and dressing into a large bowl and serve immediately.

CURRY SALAD

Ingredients
2 tspns curry powder
¼ cup lime juice
3 tblspns olive oil
salt and pepper

250g (7oz) green beans trimmed and cut in half
1 small cauliflower de-stalked and separated
1 cup frozen corn
1 Aloe vera leaf blended

Method
Toast curry powder in dry frying pan for about 1 minute. To make the vinaigrette, mix lime juice, curry powder, salt, pepper and Aloe vera into a small bowl. Steam cauliflower and beans for about 5 minutes then rinse under cold water. Once the veggies have cooled, toss them together with the vinaigrette and serve.

CRAB SALAD

Ingredients
4 handful mixed lettuce
1 cucumber
1 capsicum
1 cup of sweet corn
4 boiled eggs

Salad Dressing
3 spoonfuls mayonnaise
1 Aloe vera leaf blended
fresh basil
1 carrot
250g (9oz) crab meat

Method
Chop mixed lettuce, finely chopped carrot cucumber capsicum, chop boiled egg and add corn and finely chopped crab meat, blend up mayonnaise, Aloe vera juice and finely chopped basil and stir into salad.

Almond-Broccoli Coleslaw

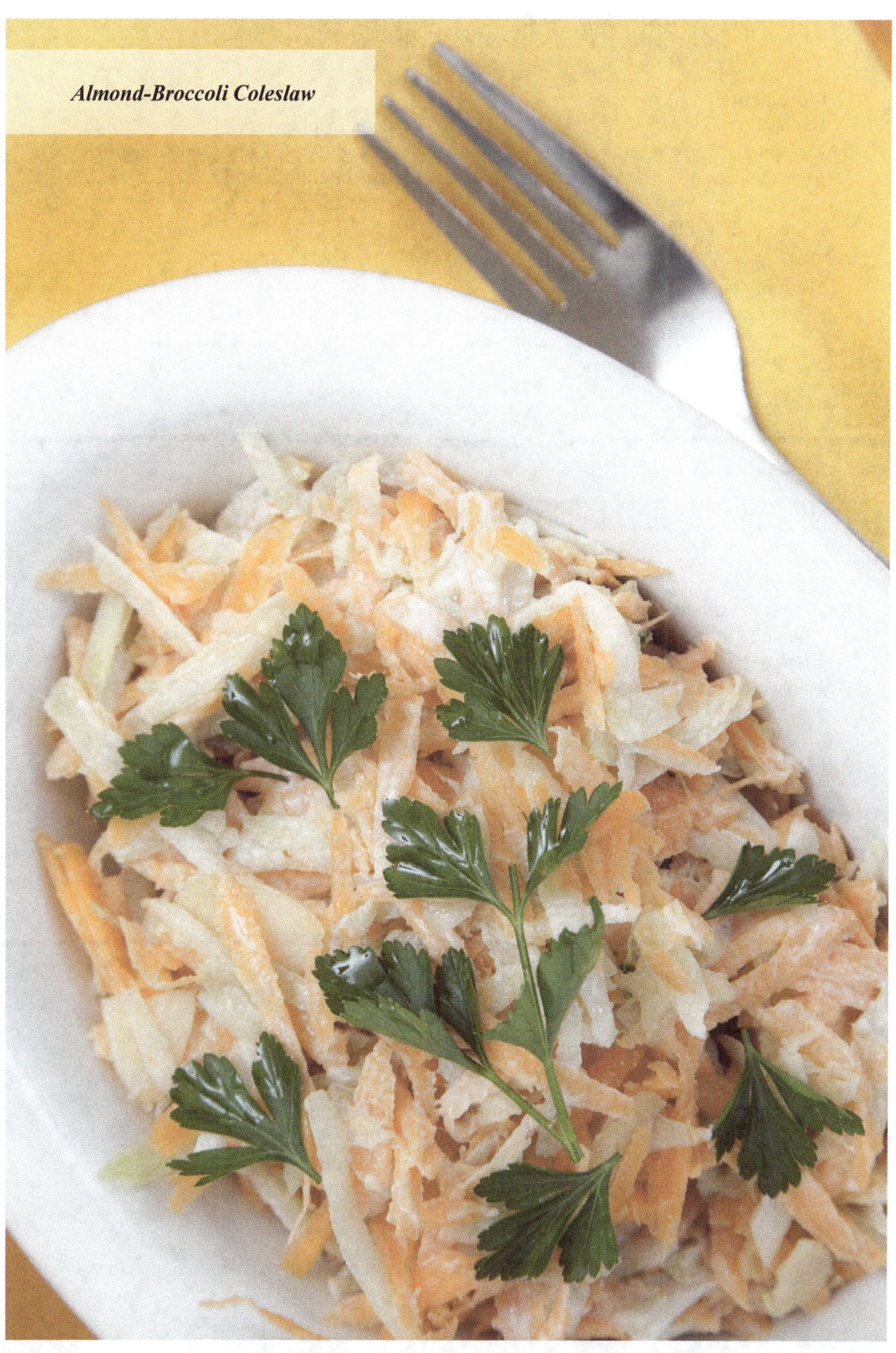

RASPBERRY AND AVOCADO SALAD

Ingredients

1 avocado
1 tblspn raspberry vinegar
1 tspn sesame oil
1 tspn honey
1 Aloe vera leaf blended

1 punnet raspberries
4 cups lightly packed watercress sprigs
2 tblspns light olive oil
1 tspn mixed herbs

Method

Remove the avocado from the skin and dice and place in a bowl on top of watercress add raspberries. Blend vinegar, oils, honey, mixed herbs and Aloe vera. Gently mix with Avocado and raspberries.

SNOW PEAS AND RADISH SALAD

Ingredients

175g (6oz) trimmed snow peas
1 bunches of radishes
1 tspn sesame oil
1 tblspn balsamic vinegar
1 Aloe vera leaf blended

2 cucumbers
1 tblspn sesame seeds (toasted)
2 tspns soy sauce
1 tspn honey
salt and pepper to taste

Method

Cook snow peas for 2-3 minutes. Drain and place over cold running water for a few minutes. Blend gel from the Aloe leaf vinegar honey soy sauce oil until smooth. Combine snow peas thinly sliced cucumber and radishes sesame seeds and add vinaigrette.

PINEAPPLE SALAD

Ingredients

½ pineapple
1 cucumber
1 cup of coriander
drizzle of balsamic vinegar

1 purple onion
1 chilli
mixed lettuce
1 Aloe vera leaf blended

Method

Finely chop all ingredients, sprinkle on the basil, salt and pepper. Blend Aloe vera gel and vinegar and drizzle over salad

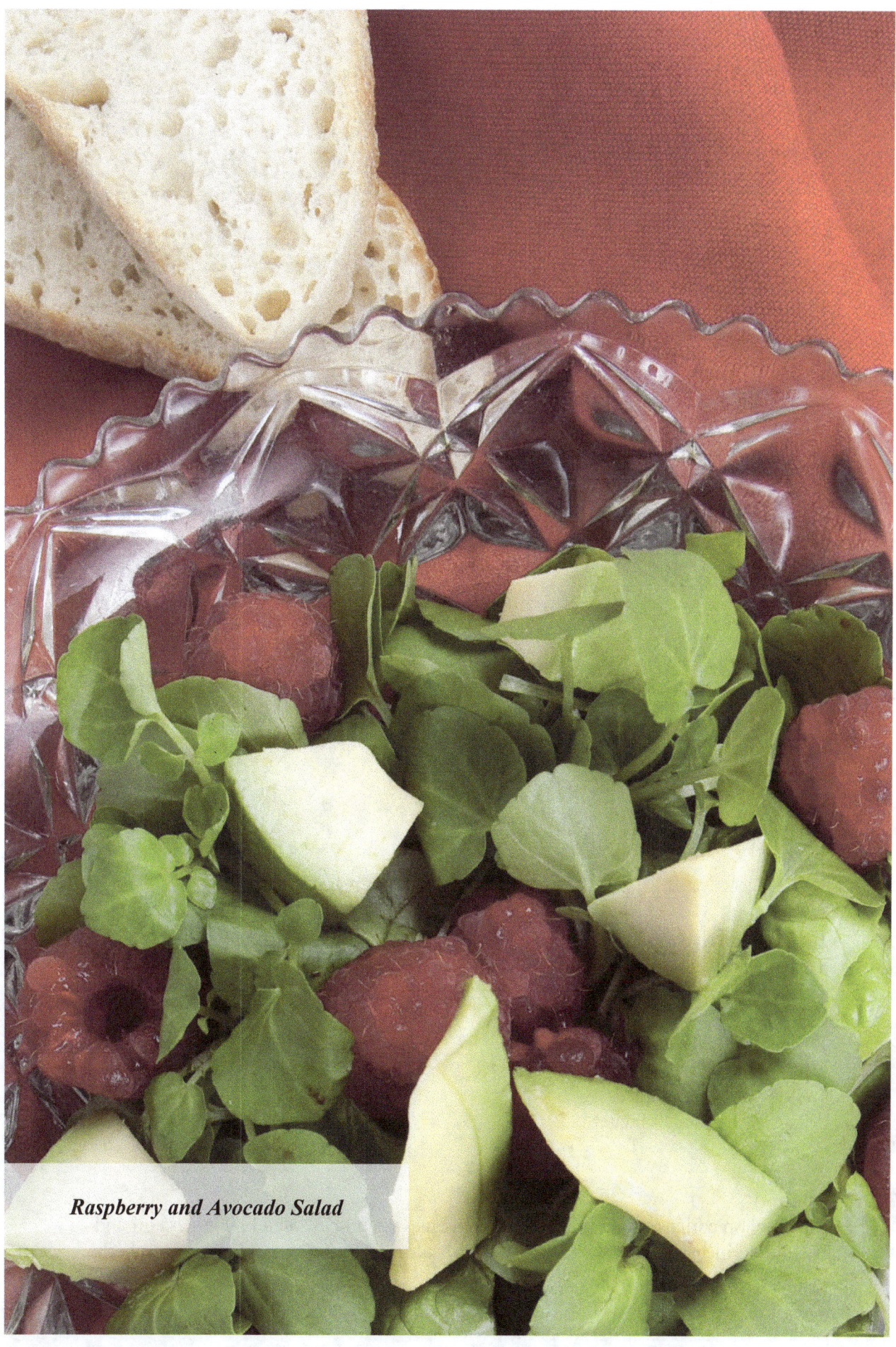

Raspberry and Avocado Salad

DUCK AND PEAR SALAD

Ingredients
watercress and rocket
smoked duck breast
2 pears sliced
8 cooked tips
1 punnet raspberries or blueberries
2 tspns mixed herbs
1 Aloe vera leaf blended
1 tblspn sesame oil
1 tblspn balsamic vinegar

Method
Place watercress and rocket on the plate, thinly slice the cooked duck and pears and also place asparagus and raspberries or blueberries. Blend Aloe vera ,oil, vinegar and mixed herbs. Drizzle over the plate.

JULIANNE SALAD

Ingredients
1 handful fresh coriander
3 tblspns olive oil
1 carrot
1 apple
1 cucumber
salt, pepper and mixed herbs
1 Aloe vera leaf blended
drizzle of balsamic vinegar

Method
Finely chop coriander and grate carrot apple and cucumber, blend Aloe vera oil and balsamic vinegar drizzle over salad and add salt and pepper to taste and mixed herbs.

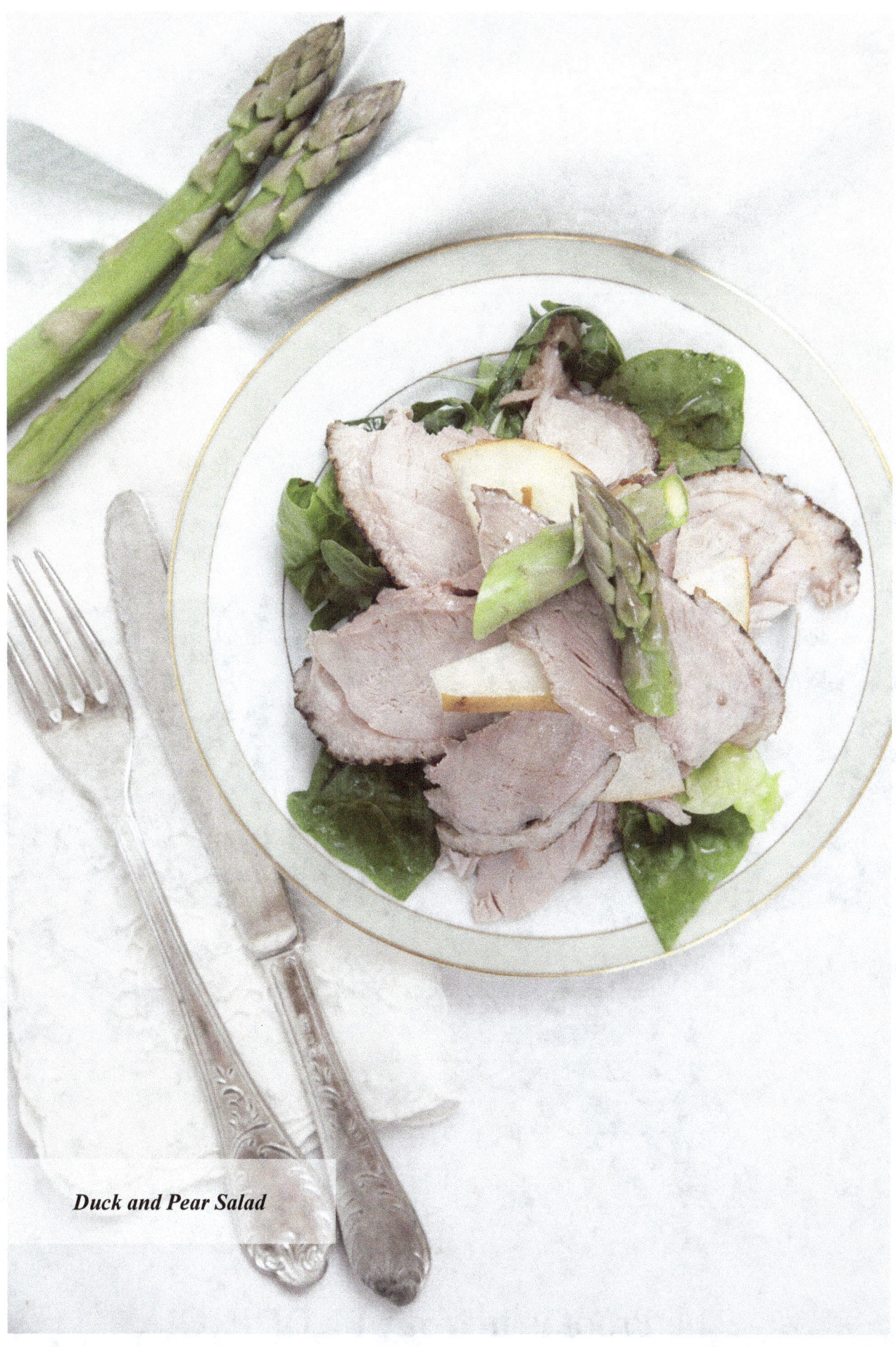

Duck and Pear Salad

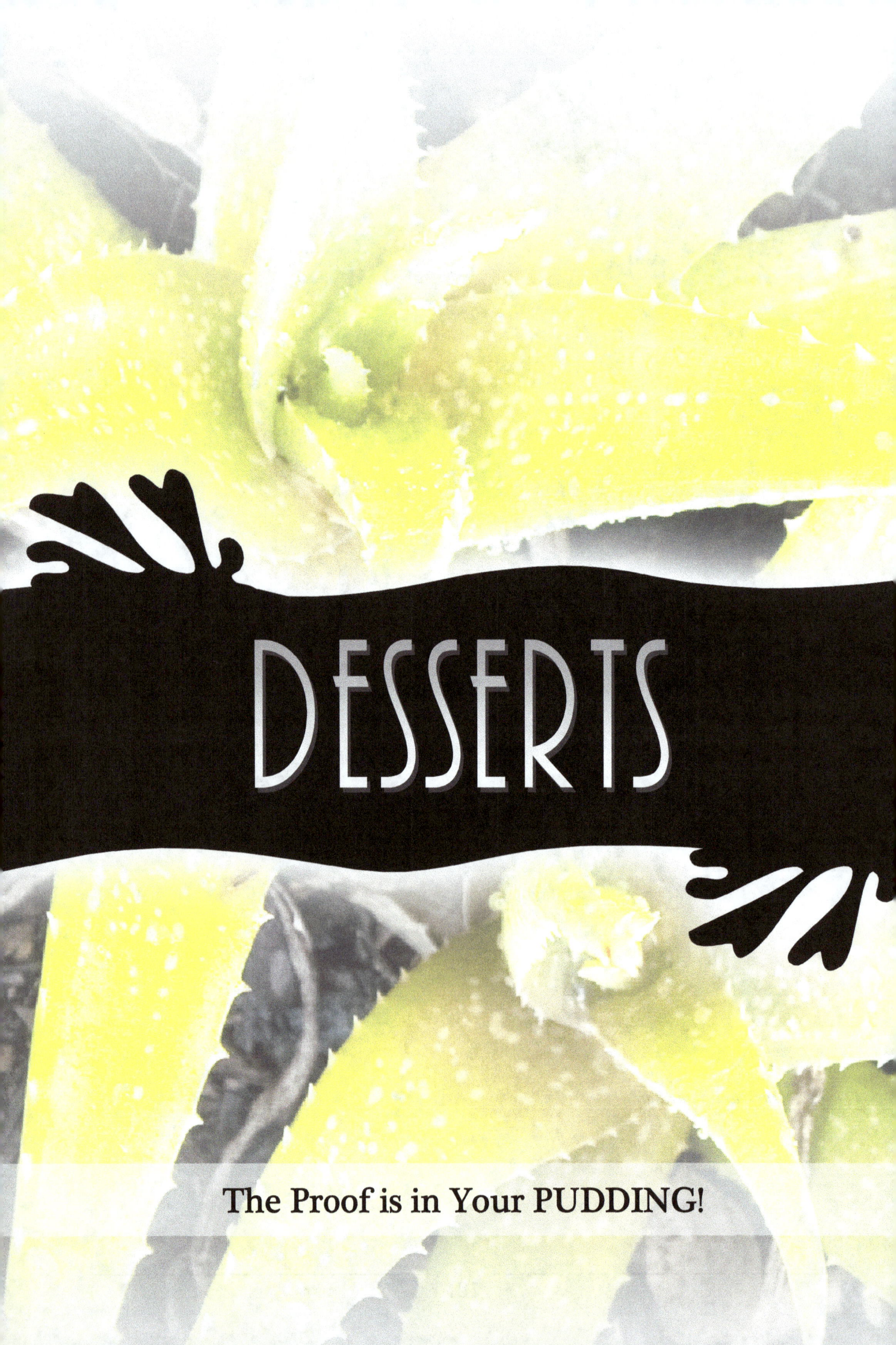

DESSERTS

The Proof is in Your PUDDING!

BLACKBERRY INDULGENCE

Ingredients

2 cups blackberries
1 cup low fat evaporated milk
½ cup caster sugar
1 Aloe vera leaf blended

Method

Puree the 2 cups of blackberries and the caster sugar in a food processor with the gel of one Aloe leaf. Whip the evaporated milk in a medium bowl until soft peaks form. Fold into the blackberry mix. Place into four serving bowls or glasses and put into the fridge for 30 minutes.

CITRUS SALAD IN ELIXIR

Ingredients

1 cup water
1 tblspn cinnamon
1 vanilla bean, split and scraped
1 orange peeled cubed
4 passion fruits
½ tspn caster sugar
1 tblspn ginger
½ lemon juice and whole peel
1 apple cubed
1 Aloe vera leaf blended

Method

Put water in a saucepan with sugar, star anise, cinnamon crushed ginger, vanilla beans scraped, peel and lemon juice. Simmer for 15-20 minutes. And then allow to cool. Remove peel. Cube all the fruits and place into a bowl. Pour Elixir over the fruit and refrigerate. Just before serving mix the Blended Aloe vera into the bowl and mix thoroughly.

FRUIT SALAD WITH YOGHURT AND LIME SAUCE

Ingredients

¼ water melon cubed
½ rock melon cubed
¼ honeydew melon cubed
½ cup seedless red and green grapes
½ cup pineapple pieces
1 cup plain low-fat yoghurt
2 tblspns reduced fat yoghurt
2 tblspns reduced fat sour cream
2 tblspns honey
1 tblspn lime juice
pinch of ginger
1 Aloe vera leaf blended

Method

Cube and place all the fruit into a bowl and refrigerate. Mix the yoghurt, sour cream, honey, lime juice and a pinch of ginger in a small bowl and refrigerate. Serve the fruit in individual bowls. Remove the yoghurt sauce and mix the blended Aloe vera into the sauce well serve in a separate bowl and let people serve themselves.

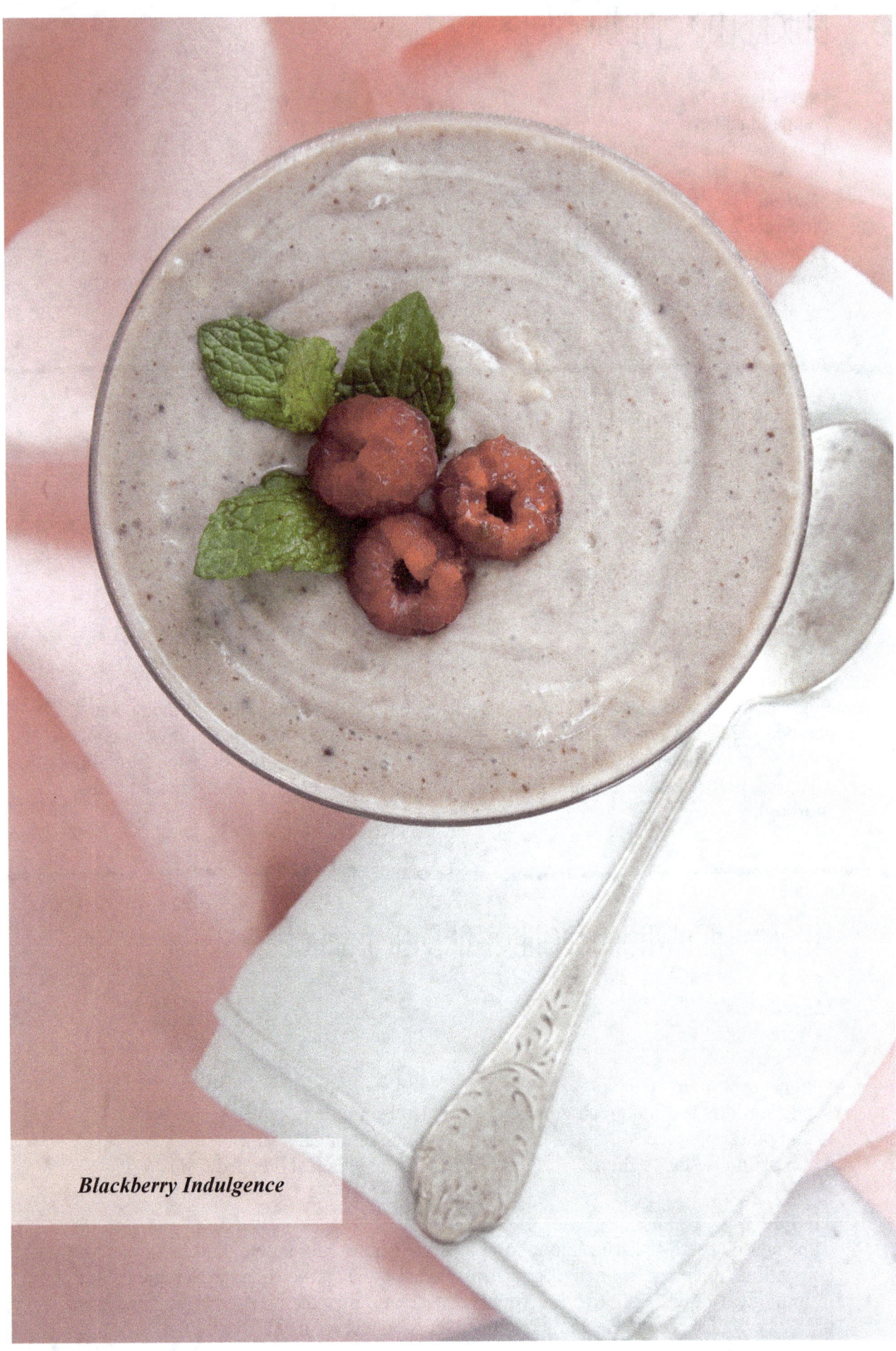

Blackberry Indulgence

FRUIT STICKS DIPPED IN YOGHURT/CHOCOLATE

Ingredients

6 wooden sticks or skewers
6 kiwi fruit
1 Aloe vera leaf blended
1 tub dipping chocolate
1 punnet strawberries
½ watermelon
1 tub vanilla yoghurt

Method

Cube the fruit and de leaf the strawberries, place the fruit on the skewers and put on a plate ready to serve. Put some yoghurt into a bowl and mix the blended Aloe vera into it thoroughly. Put chocolate into a separate bowl. This is a great favourite for the kids and you can use all types of fruit and yoghurt you wish. It is fun and really healthy, the chocolate is high in unsaturated fats but the occasional indulgence is nice.

KIWI FRUIT AND RICOTTA CREAM

Ingredients

¼ cup caster sugar
8 kiwi fruit peeled and sliced
½ cup low fat ricotta cheese
2 tspns lime zest
1 Aloe vera leaf blended
¼ cup lime juice
½ tspn grated lime zest
2 tblspns reduced fat sour cream
1 tblspn honey

Method

Place the sugar and lime into a bowl with the kiwi fruit and refrigerate for at least 30 minutes. In a jug put the grated lime zest, ricotta, sour cream, honey and Aloe vera and blend. Serve the kiwi fruit with its syrup in bowls, with the ricotta cream on top and cut the lime zest into fine shavings and decorate.

STRAWBERRIES IN GINGER/MINT SYRUP WITH VANILLA YOGHURT

Ingredients

400 gram (14oz) fresh strawberries

Mint Syrup

1 cup water
1 tblspn ginger
2 strips lemon peel
1 cinnamon stick
1 tspn mint leaves
1 tspn honey

Yoghurt

800g (28oz) plain low fat yoghurt
1 vanilla pod split and scraped
½ tspn honey
1 blended Aloe vera leaf

Syrup

Mix water, ginger, lemon peel, cinnamon, mint and honey. Bring to boil reduce heat and simmer until liquid reduces by half, strain liquid and allow to cool then add blended Aloe vera gel. thoroughly.

Yoghurt

Mix honey with a small amount of warm water to the honey, then add yoghurt and vanilla and mix until all combined. Place yoghurt in bowls topped with strawberries and syrup.

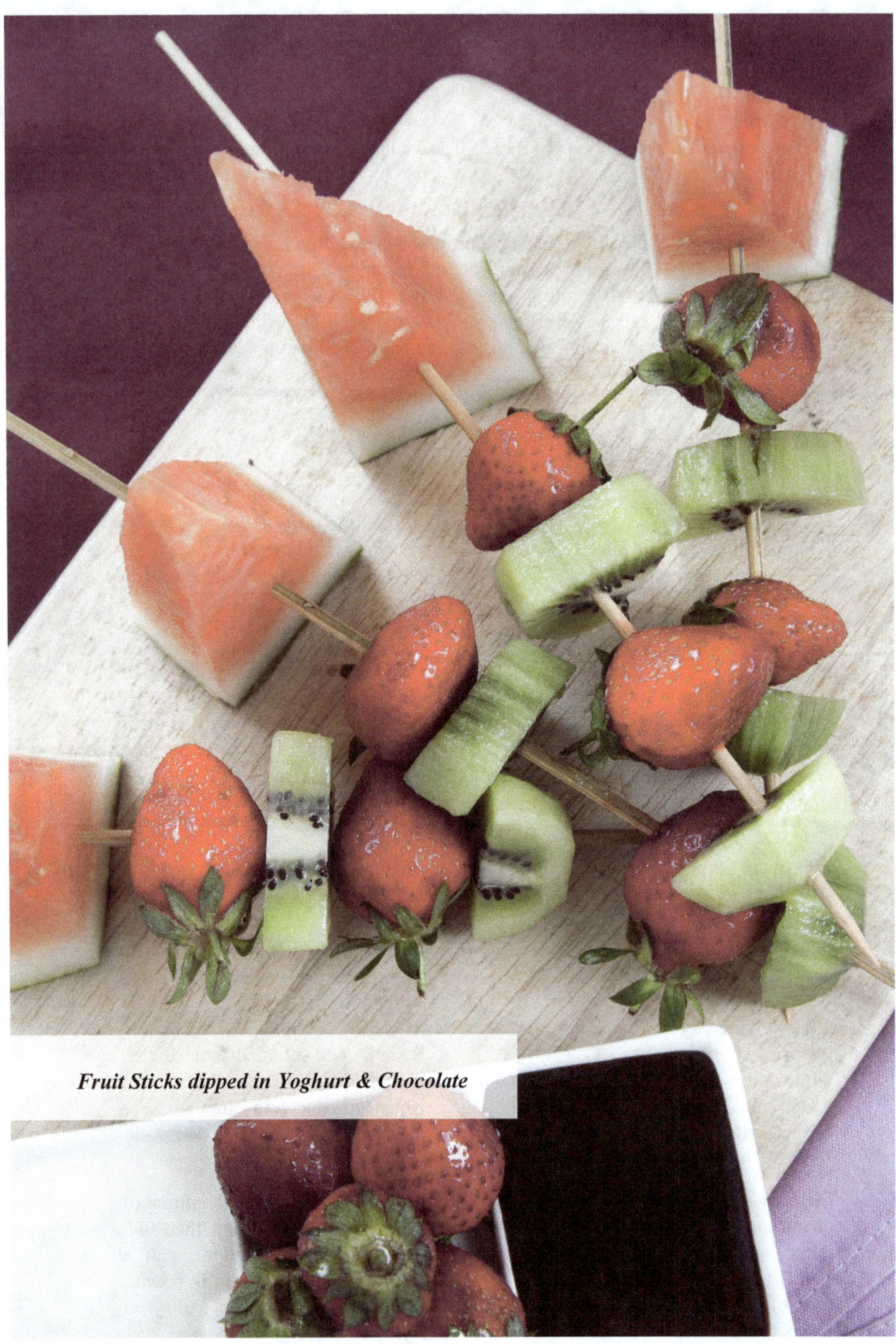

Fruit Sticks dipped in Yoghurt & Chocolate

CHOCOLATE RIPPLE CAKE

(Special occasions only. Kids especially love to make these two cakes and, with no baking, it is very easy for them)

Ingredients
1 bottle cream
1 packet of chocolate ripple biscuits
2 drops vanilla essence
2 tblspns sugar

Method
Place cream sugar and vanilla essence in a bowl and beat until cream is whipped. Get a butter knife and smother cream on one side of the biscuit, get another biscuit and smother cream on it, then place the un-creamed side onto the first biscuit, continue until all biscuits are creamed. Then smother the log with cream, cover and place into the fridge over night to soften the biscuit and make it soft and moist. You can sprinkle with grated chocolate if you wish but it is already very rich.

ICE CREAM CAKE

(Only for special occasions)

Ingredients.
1 tub Neapolitan ice-cream (three colours in one tub)
1 bottle cream
2 tblspns sugar
2 drops vanilla essence
1 bag mixed lollies
1 bag marshmallow pieces
1 small block milk chocolate

Method
Turn the tub of ice cream upside down and remove the plastic. If ice cream is showing signs of melting, place into the freezer for fifteen minutes. Whip cream, sugar and vanilla together and cover the ice cream. Place chopped lollies and chocolate pieces all over the cake and quickly put it into the freezer or serve immediately.

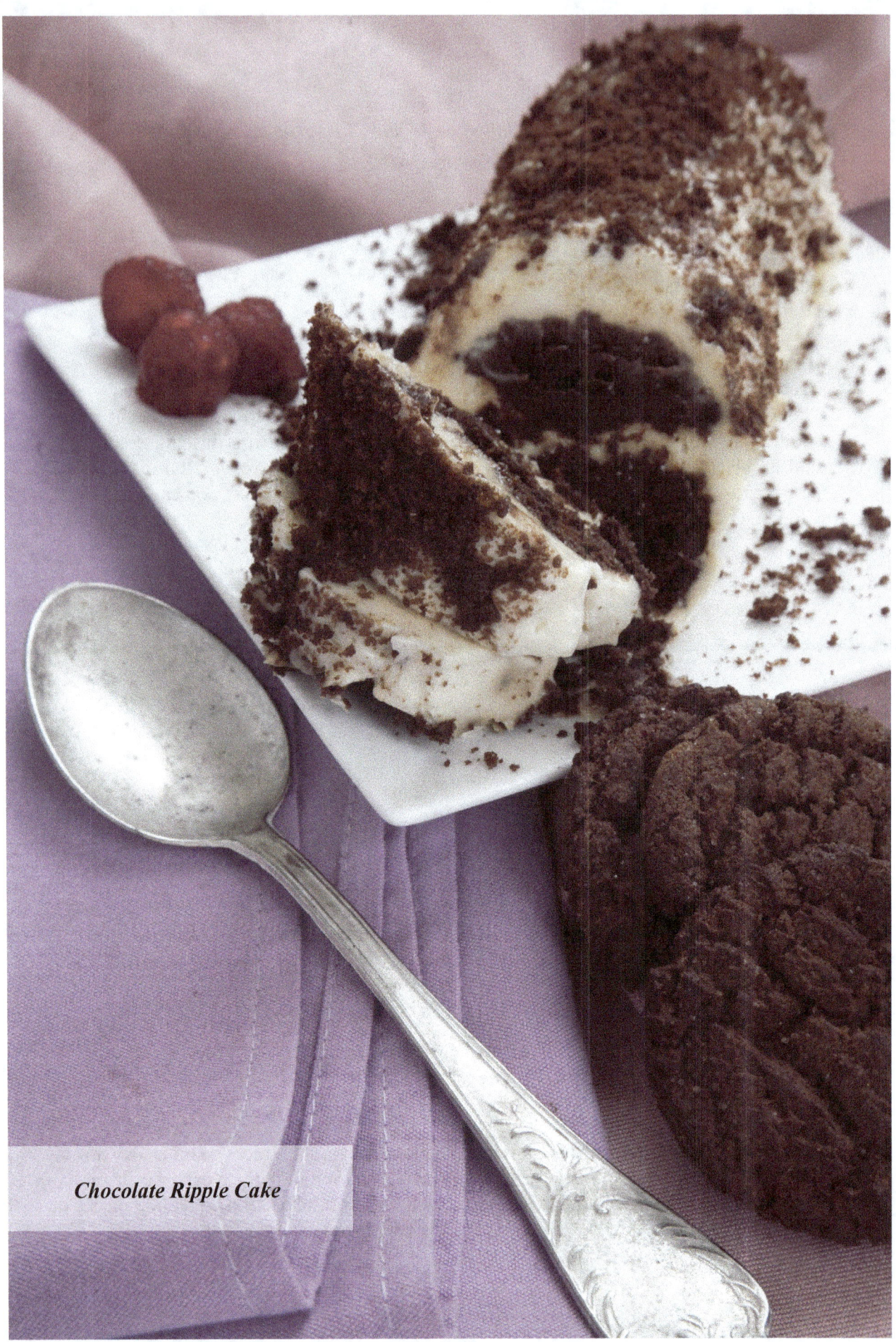

Chocolate Ripple Cake

MIRACLE DOGGIE TREATS

Ingredients
2 cups oat bran
2 cups plain flour
200ml (15fl oz) gravy
1 Aloe vera leaves

Method
When you are making a roast chicken make enough gravy for this recipe. Then blend Aloe vera gel and gravy together in a jug. Knead dough. Cut into small shapes with a bone cutter. Place on an oven tray and cook at 200°C (400°F) for 15- 20 minutes or until golden brown. Once they have cooled down place 1/2 a dozen into plastic resealable bags keep one bag out for the dog and place the others in the freezer as they have no preservative and can go off quickly.

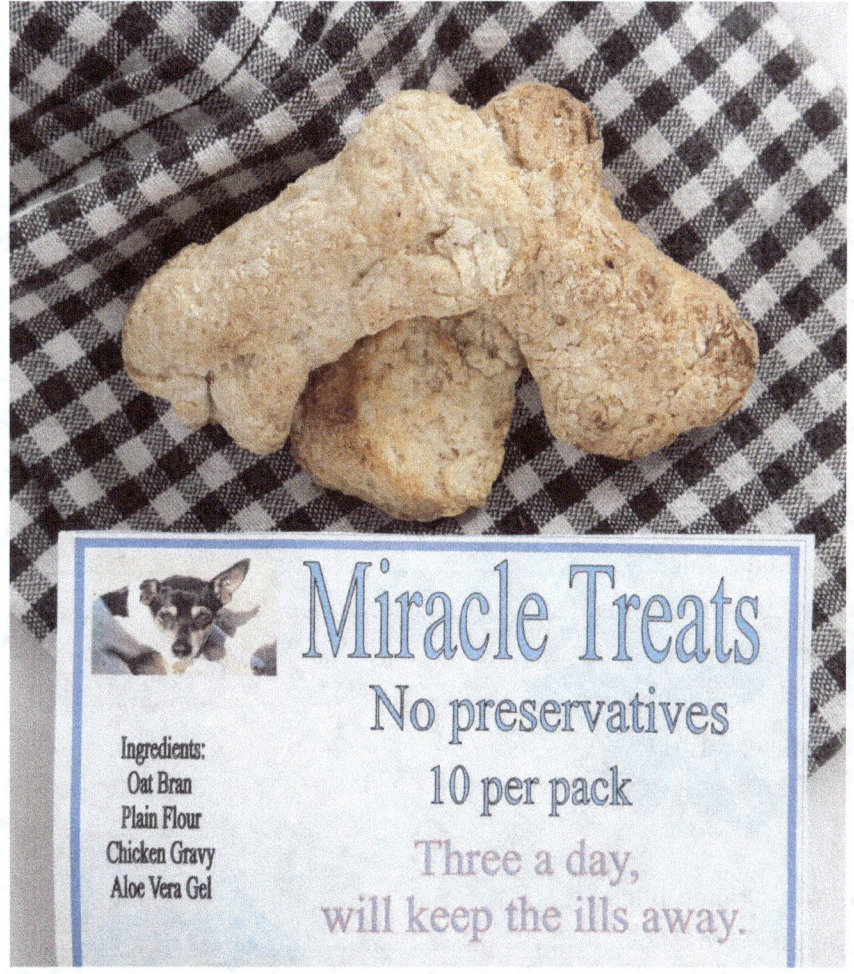

RECIPE INDEX

A

Almond-Broccoli Coleslaw 96
Aloe Power Drink 11
Aloe vera Juice..v, 10
Apple Al Smoothie 28
Apple and Carrot Juice..12
Apple Pork Steaks and Bean Salsa 85
Asparagus and Apple 12
Avocado and Mango Sauce 31

B

Ban-Mango Smoothie 26
BBQ Prawns..60
BBQ Salad Mix..94
BBQ Seafood Sticks 58
Beanie Juice 18
Beef and Veggie Salad...71
Beef and Veggie Wraps 73
Beef Curry...71
Beef Stir Fry..69
Beet in the Juice 16
Berry and Mandarin Glazed Breasts 49
Berry Smoothie 28
Blackberry Indulgence 103
BOk choy Stir Fry Pork 83

C

Carrot-Orange Juice 15
Cheesy Corn Chowder 39
Cherry TomatoEs with stuffed Pesto 33
Chicken and Bacon Stir Fry...47
Chicken and Five Bean Wrap 35
Chicken Meatloaf..51
Chicken Parmigiana..51
Chilli baby Octopus 56

Chinese Chicken Noodles 53
Chocolate Ripple Cake 107
Citrus and Pine Nut Salad 90
Citrus Salad in Elixir 103
Crab Salad 96
Crab Sauté 62
Cream of Broccoli Soup 37
Creamy Chicken Soup 35
Creamy Vegetable Soup 37
Curry Salad 96

D

Duck and Pear Salad 100

E

Egg Salad 92
Eggplant Dip 33

F

Fruit Salad with Yoghurt and Lime Sauce 103
Fruit Sticks dipped in Yoghurt/chocolate 105
Fruity Veggie Drink 17

G

Grilled Chicken in Chilli and Mango Sauce 43
Grilled Chicken in Yoghurt Marinade 45

H

Happy Mango Juice 21

I

Ice Cream Cake 107
Irish Stew 80

J

Juicy Beet 24
Julianne Salad 100

K

Kiwi Fruit and Ricotta Cream 105

L

Lamb in Mint Sauce Marinade 78
Lamb in Sage and Tarragon Paste 76
Lamb Meatballs 78
Lamb Tenderloins in Orange Marinade 76
Lemon and Chilli Calamari Barbequed 60
Lemon and Honey Drink 14
Lemon Grass Pork Skewers 87
Lettuce and Tomato Vinaigrette 90

M

Mandy Al Smoothie 28
Minestrone Soup 37
Miracle Doggie Treats 109
Mixed Seafood Soup 41
Moroccan Beef 67
Mushroom Salad 92
Mussels in Herb and Garlic Sauce 58

O

Orange and Basil Veal Bake 67
Orange and Sesame Salad 90

P

Pasta Salad 94
Peach on the go 26
Pine a Melon Crush 23
Pineapple Salad 98
Pine-Berry Zing 19
Pine-Carrot Zing 20
Pine-Orange Smoothie 26
Pork and Bean Chilli 83
Pumpkin and Apple Soup 35

R

Radish Salad	92
Raspberry and Apple Icy	12
Raspberry and Avocado Salad	98
Roast Chicken with Vegetables	53
Roast Pork with Stuffed Apple and Rosemary	87
Roasted Rack of Lamb in Honey	80
Rocket and Citrus Salad	94
Rosemary and Garlic stuffed Lamb	76
Rosemary and Orange Sauce over Chicken	49

S

Satay Chicken	45
Scallop and Cherry Tomato Sauté	62
Snow Peas and Radish Salad	98
Stir Fry Chicken and Cashews	47
Strawberries in Ginger/Mint Syrup with Vanilla Yoghurt	105
Stuffed Pork with Apple Sauce	85

T

Tahini Dip	31
Tandoori Chicken Ribs	43
Thai Beef Burger	73
Thai Prawn Soup	39
Toasted Bread and Garlic Mushrooms	33
Tropical Blended Juice	22

V

Veal in Orange and Basil Sauce	69
Veggies and Peanut Dip	31

TESTIMONIAL

My grandfather used to drink Aloe vera, he put it on his sores and cuts they healed straight away, also applied it to sunburn for instant relief. As he got older his hair fell out and he was very bald so he tried rubbing it on his head and if I didn't see it for myself I would not have believed it, but his hair grew back it was not thick but it covered his head.

From Lyn Poole
Traralgon
Vic

TESTIMONIAL

I'm a 62 year old dialysis patient. I have had total kidney failure for four years now. Before I was introduced to Aloe vera, I experienced, severe pain, muscle spasms, cramps, headaches, nausea, during and after my treatment. These after effects of dialysis were debilitating and caused many emergency room visits and hospital stays.

Some time ago I was introduced to the wonderful effects of Aloe vera, infused juice and foods. I was taught how to prepare the recipe that improved my life tremendously. Now I experience less medication, less aches and pains, no emergency room or hospital stays, since I started using the stuff. Further investigation revealed my nausea was due to an ulcer, which the Aloe vera has taken care of as well.

My doctor and dietician is amazed at my lab (blood-test) numbers and over all health improvement. I have actually regained some kidney function. With more improvement I'm hoping to forego my upcoming transplant.

What's the formula? I only do the juice everyday and the foods once in awhile. I started on straight Aloe vera and orange juice, but changed to Aloe vera and cranberry, because the acid in the orange irritated my stomach. The cranberry juice and Aloe vera worked out just fine, and I showed great improvement for several weeks.

Then I was asked to try what I consider the "Holy Grail". It's a full mix of fresh green bean, fresh carrots, cut apple and of course Aloe vera. I use apple juice to mix it in my kitchen blender. I've been doing this for quite some time now and my general health continues to improve.

I'm hooked I won't stop, it's the greatest. With Aloe I'm living a better quality of life. I wish I had learned of Aloe sooner. After two months of drinking Aloe vera every day the tablet intake has shrunk by half.

WALTER HOWARD   Daytona Beach, Florida

Continued overleaf...

...from prior page...

A further six months on after the kidney transplant -

My blood levels are only tested monthly and so far so good. At my annual major whole body testing in February, they gave me a bone density test and found I needed another drug (age related) and vitamin D level was low (I get little or no natural sunlight), a supplement took care of that.

Since the transplant I have lost 20lbs and become very "Buff," due to the vigorous workouts I do 3 times a week and swimming in between. I never felt better in my adult life. First time in my life I ever owned a "Muscle Shirt" LOL

I drink my Aloe daily and rub the split leaf over my face and body which makes me look and feel radiant inside, and out. All the plants are doing great and one or two are producing babies.

Have a great day for the rest of it and a wonderful restful night.

WALTER

A few months further on -

I'm now 63 and for a few years I suffered with mild arthritis, in the neck and fingers. I also had stiffness and morning pain in other parts of my body. I increased my daily intake of Aloe mix with fresh fruit juice (Whole Fruit blended with the Aloe in a blender) to twice a day. I now have no morning pain, which before, required pain medication from time to time. I haven't needed any pain meds since I started this routine. The extra Aloe seems to lubricate the joints to re-leave the effects of the arthritis.

The other out come I've noticed, last Feb. all my doctors released me except for routine check ups. With my body being in a digressed state, I started an exercise program. Stretching first, then moderate exercise. My body started to tone up, but when I went to the two a day Aloe dose, my energy level increased and I started to build muscle. Now I do a full body building workout five or six times a week. I'm a new man, full of vigor and in the best shape since my 20's. I owe my new life style and medical state to you, Angie. (my new friend thanks you too:) You can add these latest facts about aloe to my testimony. I will be forever grateful, thank you Angie

WALTER

From Mt. Baldy to the Amazon Rain Forest

I was introduced to the wonders of the aloe vera plant about 8 months ago. At the time I had a perfectly shaped skating rink perched on top and to the back of my head. It's called a standard male baldness pattern. I just called it depressing.

When I began to help Angie with the production of her cookbook and read some of the testimonials, I asked if she had gotten any testimonials regarding hair restoration. She told me of a man who had gotten some great results by putting pure aloe vera juice right from the plane on his bald spot and it worked wonders. Of course I had to give it a try. I've been putting the juice from the aloe vera plant directly on my head for about 8 months and the results are truly remarkable. My friends tell me my new hair growth makes me look at least 10-15years younger.

Thank you Angie for helping me recapture some of my youthful appearance.

Larry Gordon

[signature]

April 30, 2009

Film Producer

TESTIMONIAL

Captain Carlton's wife Irene told me when her husband was alive he used Aloe vera to cure his skin cancers. Here is what she said.

"Cecil got skin cancers on his ears, he would rub Aloe vera on his ears. After several months the cancers slowly shrank until they were totally gone."

Irene said that he used the Aloe vera when he was a pilot over forty years ago.

Airline Pilot

TESTIMONIAL

I thought my little doggy was a dead duck.

My little black mini-schnauzer Fancy got sick on the weekend. Schnauzers often have a sensitive tummy and she is no exception. It was late on Friday evening and she started throwing up. I didn't think too much about it at the time because she just does that every once in a while. She didn't feel any better on Saturday and wouldn't eat. Come Sunday she had diarrhoea. I was really getting worried and afraid she would dehydrate - she is so little, still with no appetite and not drinking any water.

At about 4 am Monday morning I woke up to her pooping blood. It was just awful and I was really scared, I scooped her up and took her to the after-hours vet up the road about 20 miles. They gave her a shot and calmed her tummy down and I brought her back home. I wanted to take her to her own doggy doctor as soon as they opened. Her doggy doctor gave me no hope, but he was going to run some tests and put her on IV fluids for the day and I was able to pick her up at 5 pm. It was a horrible day, I just knew she was gone. She was 9 years old at the time.

The test came back okay, thank God, it wasn't her pancreas. She was still miserable, listless, and wouldn't eat that night. Then Angie told me about putting Aloe in her food and how to do it. I just happened to have a great big Aloe plant out back, so on Tuesday I cooked some brown rice and mixed the rice water and Aloe juice together and got her to drink a little of it. I did this several times throughout the day and by evening she was ready for some of the nice soft rice with Aloe in it. She seemed to know it was helping her.

She rested comfortably that night and Wednesday morning when I got up she was ready to eat some real doggy food and running around like a puppy, as if nothing had happened! It was unbelievable. She gave the mailman his usual greeting and I knew it was over. What a relief. I know and so does Fancy that she would not have recovered so quickly if not for the Aloe mixture. Now we use it for maintenance doses as she still has a sensitive tummy and we sure don't want to go thru that again. I am eternally grateful to Auntie Angie for the good advice that helped bring my little girl back from the brink of death and I will never ever be without an Aloe plant!

Sharon Sellers, US

MAXINE'S DOG ATTACK

Maxine was attacked by a blue heeler dog, he bit her neck and her chest she also had several puncture marks from teeth bites on her ribs and stomach. I bathed her wounds

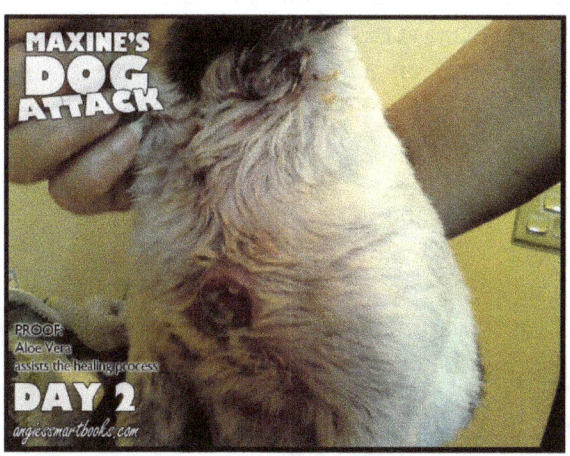

three times a day and put pieces of Aloe vera leaves over the two major wounds and held them in place with bandages. The top left picture was taken a day later and the wounds were infected from the dog's teeth. The second picture was taken six days after the attack and her wounds were clean and the swelling around the bites is just the way the Aloe vera helps it to heal up, yes the Aloe keeps the wound moist and this seems to help it heal quicker.

By day eight the hole it self has shrunk and the depth of the bite is nearly gone. She was very itchy and tried to pull her bandages off when I was not looking, sometimes she will hide the bandage in the couch trying to bury it in the cushions. I have to continually pat her to distract her from scratching them. By day ten her wounds are nearly closed and she doesn't have to wear her bandages during the day just at night now.

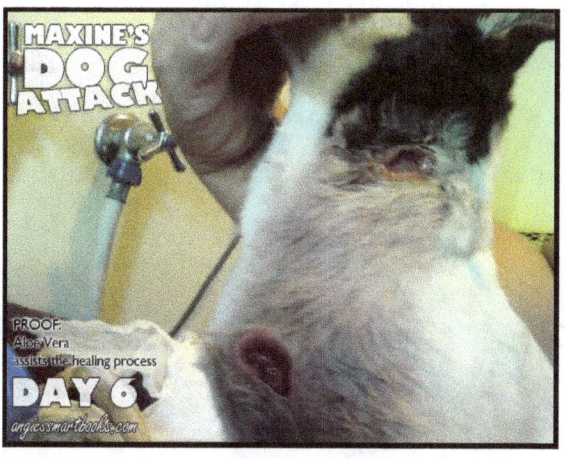

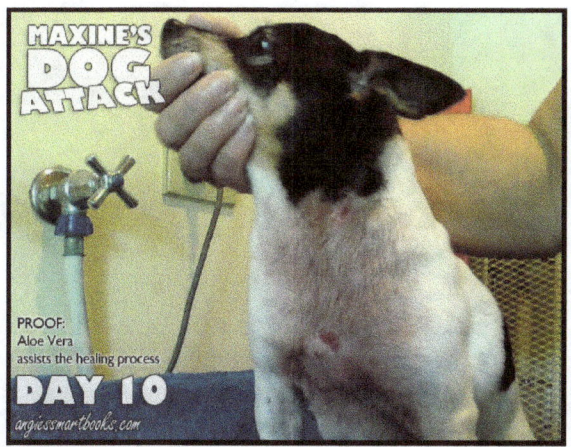

This bottom picture is of her on day ten. By day fifteen the wounds are completely healed and the scars are very minimal. Hard even for the eye to see. Aloe vera truly is a great plant. Not only saving hundreds of dollars at the vets but minimal scaring is great for all. But it is very time consuming. What we do for our loved ones even our pets.

TESTIMONIAL

I have suffered from cold sores for most of my life, but when my marriage was nearing the end I contracted herpes - one of the final gifts my ex gave me. I decided to try Aloe vera on them when they came up. I found if I put the Aloe vera on as soon as I felt its presence, the soreness would be alleviated in 24 hours, and the sore itself would go in a few days.

With continual drinking and eating of the Aloe vera I have not had a cold sore or herpes for many years now. I am sure this will also help relatively similar ailments like shingles. If you can actually slice the Aloe vera open and sit the plant on the ailment for two hours you may find the pain will go away much quicker.

This is a great way to deter the sores and even stop them from coming back as the Aloe vera has over 100 different vitamins, minerals and enzyme in it so it is very good at regenerating healthy new cells.

Angie Andrews

TESTIMONIAL

This letter is from my friend who had just woken up with shingles and its terrible pain. I suggested she try Aloe vera. Here is what she did...

> Gosh, I was so excited that I just exposed the nectar and put the wet part of the leaf right on the area. Because it is on my back it doesn't just stay there. I will have to get some medical adhesive of some kind to hold it in place. However, this morning it is not as pronounced as it was -- hopefully that will start assisting with healing immediately. The great news is I don't utilize any chemicals on the plant's just water, natural compost, and miracle grow.
>
> The first leaf I applied on soaked completely into the skin in about 2 or 3 minutes. I was checked the leaf and all of the gel was gone -- so I lightly rubbed the area of my back and it was dry. It was remarkable how fast the skin took in the healing gel and completely absorbed what was available on the first leaf. Then I put on a second much larger leaf and its nectar was gone in about 15 minutes. I guess that shows that the skin was needing the Aloe Vera properties very much; as when my skin is healthy it takes longer to absorb natural lotions to soften the skin. lol
>
> I am happy to know what this is -- I completely forgot that it is from the *Herpes Zoter* family and frankly, I am thankful that I didn't go and meet folks at those conferences and events where they could have been exposed and shared in a dose of shingles. However, anyone that doubts that I have shingles, is certainly invited to spend some quality time with me and I will certain give them a big hug!
>
> Suellis

Suellis has had aids for many years with her T-cell count in the thousands. Since she bought my cookbook over six months ago, her blood levels are now nearly back to normal, here is one more comment she emailed to me after a visit to the doctor on the first week of December 2011...

> The t-cell count is about 245 -- above 200 -- another celebration moment -- and considering that I have been hoarding the meds for some time now (not using them). The Aloe Vera sure has held things in place for a very long time - unexplainably so.
>
> Suellis

TESTIMONIAL

Dear Angie,

I feel compelled to thank you again for publishing your book Cookin' for Cures. I have been eating Aloe vera, and I feel more awesome inside and out, than I ever did before in my life!

I am insulin-dependent, a Type-1 Diabetic - For people who are unaware, I would like to point out that Type-2 Diabetes, is also known as Sugar Diabetes, and is caused by a long-period of exposure to a diet too high in sugar and saturated fats... in other words, it can be avoided - by simply eating well, and exercising. Type-1 Diabetes is an Auto-Immune disorder which often occurs to children who have experienced a series of stressful events in their life, along with an incorrect balance of sugars, fiber, fat, protein, vitamins and minerals in their diet.

I haven't always looked after myself according to the treatment outlined by the professionals. As a result, I have suffered prolonged High Blood Sugar periods which, at various times have wreaked havoc on my physical body - my body trying to rid itself of excess glucose - and even when my levels are good, my toes and groin often exhibit signs of tinea (athlete's foot).

I have been experimenting with Aloe vera as a replacement for topical creams, and as a healthful food for over five years now. My daily Aloe vera smoothie in the morning with fruit like bananas, yogurt and protein powder to cover the bitter taste.

I stopped using Aloe vera fortified sprays, creams and toothpastes because I found that using the fresh gel from the plant is so much better! I simply can't believe how healthy my teeth, gums, and everything else have become.

Simply by adding Aloe vera to my regular diet and sipping several glasses of fresh clean water daily, I find I am no longer falling asleep at my desk in the middle of the day, and not running to the bathroom with a full bladder every fifteen minutes either! I am amazed at how I can still work at my peak, despite being age 41 and having lived with Type-1 diabetes for 22 years now!

Thank-you! Thank-you! Thank-you!

Glenn T. Wallace BMM
phormulae.com